Pilates

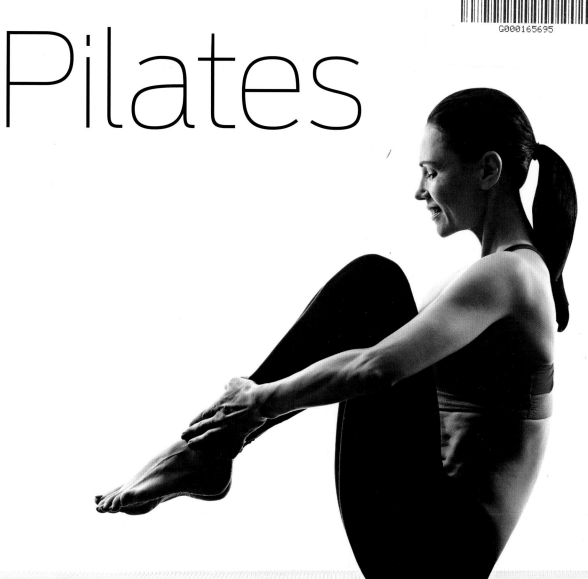

Pilates

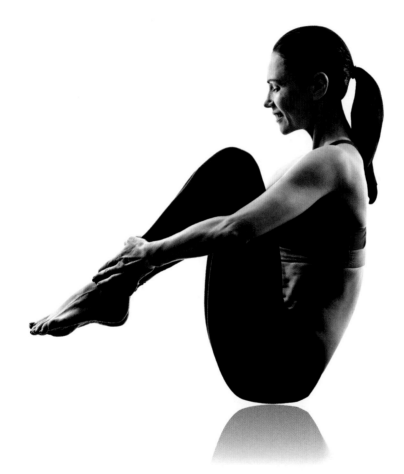

Isabel Eisen

hinkler

Published by Hinkler Books Pty Ltd 2021
45–55 Fairchild Street
Heatherton Victoria 3202 Australia
www.hinkler.com.au

hinkler

Created by Moseley Road Inc.
Editorial Director: Lisa Purcell
Art Director: Brian MacMullen
Photographer: Jonathan Conklin Photography, Inc.
Editor: Erica Gordon-Mallin
Designers: Danielle Scaramuzzo, Patrick Johnson
Author: Isabel Eisen
Model: Brooke Marrone
Nutrition writer: Cori D. Cohen, RD
Illustrator: Hector Aiza/3D Labz Animation India
Cover Design: Sam Grimmer

ISBN: 978 1 4889 2312 8

Printed and bound in China

Always do the warm-up exercises before attempting any individual exercises. It is recommended that you check with
your doctor or healthcare professional before commencing any exercise regime. While every care has been taken in
the preparation of this material, the publishers and their respective employees or agents will not accept responsibility
for injury or damage occasioned to any person as a result of participation in the activities described in this book.

Contents

Fitness for Life

Whether you focus on classical-style Pilates exercises or choose to explore new twists on the classics, Pilates offers you a rich and rewarding method to get fit and strong.

Welcome to *proActive: Pilates* and to a rewarding and invigorating exercise program. The discipline of Pilates accomplishes wonders for a wide range of people, and it can also be practiced just about anytime and anywhere.

The Pilates method

The Pilates method is a balanced, safe, and effective approach to fitness conditioning that you can begin practicing it at any age. Pilates addresses both general and specific goals—whether these goals involve work or everyday activities, sports performance, injury prevention, or "just" the need for better overall health. As a student of Pilates, you'll experience that your mindful, precise, and fluid exercising will spur and support a rapid improvement in physical stability, strength, and flexibility. Pilates helps to keep your body and mind aligned throughout your lifetime. With regular practice, you'll look great and feel amazing.

This book is a comprehensive guide to practicing Pilates at home. Classical and "beyond the classics" exercises are described and explained through photos and anatomical illustrations, so that you can more fully understand each exercise, while forming mental images of how your muscles relate to what you're doing. This versatile yet concise information will support the correct mind-body execution of each exercise.

Before you plunge into your Pilates regimen, it's important to stop for a moment and gather some information about the roots and fundamentals of the method. As you begin to explore, you'll come to understand more deeply that the Pilates method is a marvelous fitness program that enables you to sculpt your body without adding bulk and strengthen your muscles without risking injury.

We'll look at the origins of Pilates, talk about the essential principles of the system, introduce you to some very useful terms, and talk about your "powerhouse," that core of muscles that is the central focus of all Pilates work. Food and drink nurture your muscles and bones and influence your daily activities and exercise routines, so we have also included a section on nutrition.

The history of Pilates

Joseph Pilates developed the Pilates system (originally called Contrology) during the early part of the twentieth century in Germany, where he was born, and then in New York City, where he taught from 1926 to 1966. Although he was a fragile child, he eventually became an accomplished gymnast, body builder, and physical trainer, and he designed rehabilitation equipment and exercises for bedridden prisoners of war during World War II.

Inspired by philosophies embodied by yoga, Zen Buddhism, Chinese martial arts, and the ancient Greek ideal of the perfect integrated human, as well as his studies of anatomy, Joseph Pilates developed a method of exercising grounded in the connection between the body and the mind. He built his method on six primary principles: centering, control, flow, breath, precision, and concentration (see pages 10–13). Pilates, then as now, consists of exercises that flow into each other at a controlled pace, that progress from smaller to larger movements, from lying on a mat to standing on it—always with an awareness of the correct alignment of the body in space.

A new generation of Pilates

Dancers and elite athletes have long been faithful students of Pilates. In the 1980s, however, the Pilates method exploded in popularity as developments in exercise science moved quite beautifully into alignment with the methodology of Joseph Pilates. The "pain makes gain" approach to exercising was reevaluated, did a flip, and landed on its feet facing a new direction. Qualitative processes were now considered at least as important as the once all-important quantitative results. More people needed to—*wanted* to—exercise. On top of all this, the exercising population had grown to include a broad spectrum of body types and ages.

The original Joseph Pilates system of exercising, which was handed down from one generation of students and teachers to the next, still exists in classical Pilates studios around the world. Within these studios, the exercises are taught exactly as Joseph Pilates taught them, and in the same order. New-generation Pilates systems still usually include a wide selection of the original exercises, though the instructor may modify a particular exercise, or order of exercises, and incorporate new moves from related fitness disciplines.

Health and fitness

Joseph Pilates' Contrology has long held a respected place among physical therapists and other healthcare professionals. Pilates helps the healthy to remain healthy, strong, supple, and physically alert. Targeted programs focus on athletic conditioning, post-rehabilitation conditioning, prenatal and postnatal conditioning, lower-back pain relief, and aging issues, as well as exercises for surviving an ordinary days spent in front of a computer or coping with too many hours stuck behind a steering wheel.

This book focuses on mat training. Pilates mat exercises require only a floor mat and are designed so that the body uses its own weight to create resistance. You can complement your mat work with special large and small apparatus that either assist movement or supply resistance. You can also easily take

Should you "reform"?

Enter almost any Pilates studio and you're bound to see rows of what look like medieval torture devices: bedlike frames, each with a moving platform attached to springs and pulleys and weights with foot bars and handles. Don't fear: this complex bit of machinery won't hurt you. It is known as the reformer—a piece of equipment Joseph Pilates designed himself.

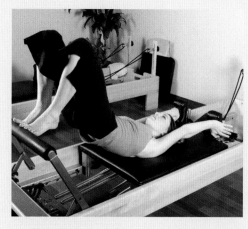

Just about any Pilates exercise performed on a mat can also be performed on the reformer. On a mat, you use your own body weight to create resistance; on a reformer, the pulleys and springs create resistance. Working against resistance is essential to Pilates. Although reformers and other specially designed Pilates equipment, like the Pilates chair, are great additions to a Pilates regimen, their size and cost (though home models are increasingly available) keep them out of reach of the typical home exerciser. But again, don't fear—you can reap great benefits whether you work on a simple mat or a complex piece of machinery.

advantage of small, portable pieces of equipment like exercise balls, stretch bands, and fitness circles, but you'll usually only find large pieces of equipment, such as the "Pilates reformer," in studios and commercial gyms.

Aligned and together

Those who practice Pilates regularly, whether at home or in a studio, usually find that they have better posture, and they feel more "aligned and together" when they leave the sanctity of the mat to tackle the activities in their daily lives. Pilates exercise also raises an awareness of the impact of deep lateral breathing, in which the breath is directed to the sides of the rib cage. This generates more efficient movement, better blood circulation, and greater energy, stamina, and vigor.

One important tenet of Pilates is that everyone should be able to benefit from it. Some of the following exercises include modifications that make them easier or more challenging, depending on your fitness level.

Remember: the quality of your movement while exercising is always more important than any quantitative striving you do along the way. Let's take a look at the Pilates Principles to understand why.

The Pilates Principles

Six concepts—centering, control, flow, breath, precision, and concentration—are often invoked as the foundations of the Pilates approach to fitness.

Spend any time with Pilates students or teachers and you're bound to hear about "centering," "control," "flow," "breath," "precision," and "concentration," often called the Pilates Principles. Contrary to what many believe, Joseph Pilates didn't directly formulate any principles. Rather, later teachers of his method distilled them from close readings of his work. This is why peppery discussion concerning which areas are essential and make up the definitive building blocks of the Pilates method is common among Pilates practitioners.

The building blocks of a method
Different schools of thought may emphasize different aspects of the Pilates method depending on their points of view, but some version of the principles is found in every Pilates style. Let's start by taking a look at centering, control, flow, breath, precision, and concentration. These concepts are interdependent and focusing on one of them really means that the others are right there, too.

A working knowledge of the principles will help infuse your practice with a mind-body awareness and intelligence that will speed up the effectiveness of your training while also deepening your appreciation of the workout. Use the anatomical illustrations in this book, as these visuals supplement the text and make the information more tangible.

Centering
Just about all bodily movement radiates from the "powerhouse" of strong muscles around the lumbar spine—between the bottom of the ribs and the line across the hips—into our arms and legs (see pages 14–15). Centering means bringing your awareness to this powerhouse and performing movements from this central core: your abdomen, lower back, hips, and buttocks.

Control
Control is an awareness of the what, where, why, when, and how of an exercise. Faulty posture—a misalignment of body

The Classics
Since Joseph Pilates first developed the Contrology system that eventually became Pilates, the list of Pilates exercises and variations on them has grown, and the order of presentation has shifted. In 1954, Pilates published *Return to Life*, in which he demonstrated 34 moves that now make up the "classical" canon. Many Pilates studios still teach the classical exercises and perform them in the same order that Joseph first stipulated.

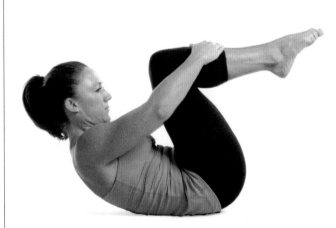

1. The Hundred
2. Roll-Up
3. Rollover
4. One-Leg Circle
5. Rolling Like a Ball
6. One-Leg Stretch
7. Double-Leg Stretch
8. Spine Stretch
9. Rocker with Open Legs
10. Corkscrew
11. The Saw
12. Swan Dive
13. One-Leg Kick
14. Double-Leg Kick
15. Neck Pull
16. The Scissors
17. Bicycle

18. Shoulder Bridge
19. Spine Twist
20. Jackknife
21. Side Kick
22. Teaser
23. Hip Twist
24. Swimming
25. Leg Pull Front
26. Leg Pull
27. Side Kick Kneeling
28. Side Bend
29. The Boomerang
30. The Seal
31. The Crab
32. The Rocking
33. Control Balance
34. Push-Up

parts—results in stress and strain on bones, muscles, joints, and ligaments. Controlled exercising develops good posture, strength, stamina, flexibility, and ease of movement, and is a tool for reestablishing our physical equilibrium when we need to find it again as, for example, after an injury. Control means finding the correct starting position before beginning an exercise (or movement), and anchoring, or stabilizing, the body in space before moving any part of it through that space. Even though most Pilates exercises don't use momentum, those that do, such as rolling and jumping exercises, are still performed with complete control. When you control your movement, you must be strong and flexible enough to allow your movement and breath to flow, grow, and lengthen.

Flow

"Flow" is a word frequently used in dance, exercise, and sports practices. Although it sounds self-evident that movement should move, not all movement flows. It's all too easy, for instance, to disrupt your flow by either "forgetting" to breathe, or by breathing in a shallow, impractical way.

Flow relates to the quality of your movement, too. Pilates exercises emphasize lengthening the body, stretching away from the center, while keeping the body compact and strong. To help you better achieve that strong, lengthened, flowing body, think of your entire exercise routine—no matter how long your practice session lasts—as a challenge to keep the flow of movement going from one exercise to the next during the transitions.

Try to create a simple, short, sequential flow of movement from the end position of one exercise to the start position of the next one.

Visual imaging

"Cueing," or using descriptive visual images of everyday concepts to stimulate correct practice, is a common Pilates teaching and learning tool, and enriches your understanding of the Pilates method during your exercise routine.

Visual imaging engages both mind and body, allowing for a better understanding of our complex human anatomical system. These images serve as metaphors that help us to use our muscles correctly with little more than a simple knowledge of muscle mechanics and function.

Some examples of these images: zipping up your front, plugging your shoulders down your back, moving from your hip creases, elongating your spine like a dart in space. As you work, you might very well find that you spontaneously think of your own visual image; don't hesitate to use it!

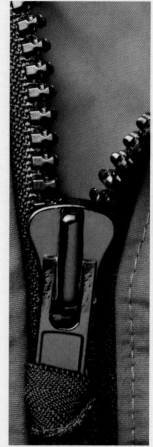

How do you know if you're "in" flow? If you feel awkward, if you feel any strain, then try again. One simple tip: let your head, your weightiest body part, follow through on a movement. Don't initiate movement with an impulse from your head and neck or you'll find yourself jerking as you pull yourself up to sitting or standing or back down to the floor. Enjoy the weight and relaxation of a heavy head, while keeping both sides of your neck long. Flow is directly connected to the breath.

Breath

A relaxed and full breathing pattern is beneficial for a healthy—efficient and energized—daily lifestyle, keeping you physically alert and generally feeling good. Most of us take breathing for granted and don't focus on how we breathe. We usually breathe shallowly, filling up the top of our lungs and not thinking about our true lung capacity. The expression of strong feelings, such as crying, laughing, and howling (try it!) uses the lungs' full capacity, and—not surprisingly—involves our powerhouse core muscles.

In the Pilates system, you breathe in deeply through your nose and expand your lower rib cage toward your sides (laterally) and fully into your back. When you exhale through your mouth, your rib cage relaxes downward compactly, as if you were snapping together two sides of a tightly fitting shirt. Your spine should remain flexible, though, with a sensation of lengthening all the time.

Each Pilates exercise has a specific breathing pattern. It can take time and repetitive practice before the coordination of the breathing with the actions of the exercise feels easy and natural. You'll just have to persevere and be patient; you'll get it sooner than you might think. Typically, exhalation takes place during the most arduous part of an exercise and inhalation on the preparation and return parts of the exercise. Never hold your breath because you're so busy focusing on the exercise sequence. Once you feel comfortable with an exercise, add the breathing pattern.

Precision

While performing exercises, precision makes it possible to move forward rapidly and develop an intuitive understanding of each one's purpose. Think about starting correctly and ending correctly and being able to trace in your mind (and later in your body, too) all those details of the small flowing segments that create the whole movement. The more you practice in a precise and mindful way, the more the Pilates method will fall into place as a natural second language.

Concentration

Concentration involves the vital mind-body connection. It's not enough to just execute a movement; you have to focus on what you're doing. You can create an image of yourself performing an exercise correctly, in proper alignment. You can build up a rhythm of sensing—with as much clarity

---

Pilates breathing

Take a look at the diagram of the human respiratory system at right, and you will notice a large dome-shaped sheet of muscle that sits beneath the lungs and extends across the bottom of the rib cage. This is the thoracic diaphragm, or simply the diaphragm.

The diaphragm separates the thoracic cavity, which shelters the heart, lungs, and ribs, from the abdominal cavity, and it also plays a major role in respiration. When we breathe, the diaphragm contracts, increasing the volume of the thoracic cavity so that air is drawn into the lungs. When the diaphragm relaxes, air is expelled.

Diaphragmatic deep breathing is a technique that helps you maximize the benefits of your Pilates practice by fully utilizing your diaphragm. Try the following exercise to learn this breathing method.

1. Lie on your back with your knees bent and one hand on your lower abdomen.
2. Inhale slowly through your nose, letting the air flow into your upper chest and then down your spine. As you inhale, you should feel your sides, lower ribs, and abdomen expand.
3. Exhale by letting the air out of your body in the opposite order in which you let it in: pull in your abdomen, ribs, and sides, and then let your chest drop as you push out the air from your nose.

During your breathing practice, be sure to keep your shoulders down and relaxed as you inhale, and concentrate on lifting your chest.

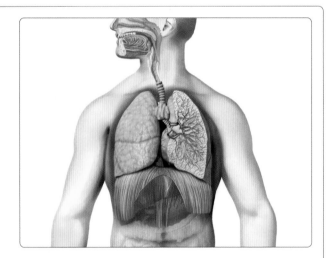

Another useful deep-breathing technique is known as lateral breathing. As the name suggest, its emphasis is sideways; in lateral breathing, you expand your breath into the back and sides of the rib cage. Directing your breath this way allows you to breathe deeply while contracting your abdominals, which gives your spine extra support during an exercise.

To practice lateral breathing, place your hands over your ribs, with your fingers pointing inward so that your middle fingers touch at your breastbone. Inhale through your nose in a deep controlled breath, allowing your rib cage to fill and expand outward, rather than upward as it would when you breathe normally. As you inhale, your fingers will part, but as you exhale, your fingertips will come together again.

as possible—the balanced muscular pathway that's going to carry that movement to completion in a strong yet melodious flow. This intertwined mind-body dialogue demands concentration. As in any performance, starting and ending correctly are no minor feats. Concentrate on start and finish precision when you perform these exercises.

Positioning

Let's concentrate for a moment on how to begin a Pilates exercise. Two basic supine positions are used in the Pilates method: neutral position and imprinted position. During any Pilates exercise, you can maintain the natural curve of your spine (neutral position), or lengthen your lumbar spine (imprinted position).

Neutral position is used during the many mat exercises, when you lie on your back in a supine position, with one or two feet on your mat. See One-Leg Circle (pages 36–37) for an example of an exercise with a neutral spine start position.

The imprinted position, on the other hand, provides extra support for your lumbar spine when you raise both feet off the mat. When imprinting, or "pressing the navel to the spine" (an image often used in Pilates teaching), the muscles of your lower back are both lengthened and strengthened and your abdominal wall is flattened. Your powerhouse is activated, muscle strength and muscle length working in collaboration and productive opposition. Both versions of the Hundred, a true Pilates classic (see pages 28–31), work from the strong imprinted position.

A quick guide to Pilates positioning

Form is all-important in Pilates, and certain positions will come up repeatedly during your workout.

neutral position: In neutral position, you maintain the natural curve of your spine—typically when lying on your back with one or both feet on the mat.

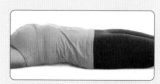

imprinted position: In imprinted position, you press your navel toward your spine. This move flattens your abdominal wall and lengthens and strengthens your lower-back muscles.

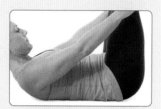

c-curve: C-curve describes the shape of your back and spine when you scoop in your stomach, stretching the muscles surrounding your spine in the process.

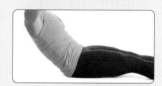

tabletop: Tabletop position is the starting point of several Pilates exercises. Lie on your back with legs raised, knees bent at a 90-degree angle. Your shins should be parallel to the ground.

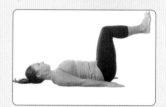

stacking: Stacking in Pilates means aligning parts of your body, such as the hips, one on top of the other, while you are positioned on your side.

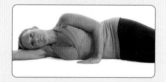

peeling the spine: Peeling the spine involves carefully rolling it vertebra by vertebra.

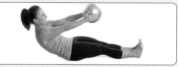

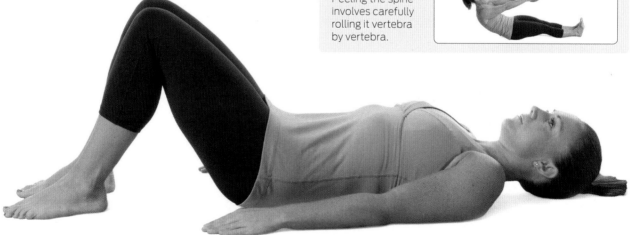

The Pilates Powerhouse

Movement radiates from the "powerhouse" of strong muscles around your lumbar spine—between the bottom of your ribs and the line across your hips—into your arms and legs.

Long before the term *core stabilization* entered the fitness lexicon, Joseph Pilates was teaching his students about the "powerhouse." He recognized that all movement emanates from the center, or core, of the body and accordingly set the primary goal of his method as strengthening that area. Strengthening the powerhouse, in effect, stabilizing the core, and a stable core provides you with a solid foundation for any movement.

The Pilates method was developed in great part as an antidote to the sedentary ways of modern life. So many of us spend days sitting at desk jobs, and our recreational activities rarely effectively challenge us physically. Joseph Pilates carefully structured a comprehensive program of stretching and strengthening exercises that work together to challenge you physically, helping you create a strong, limber body, while also focusing your mind.

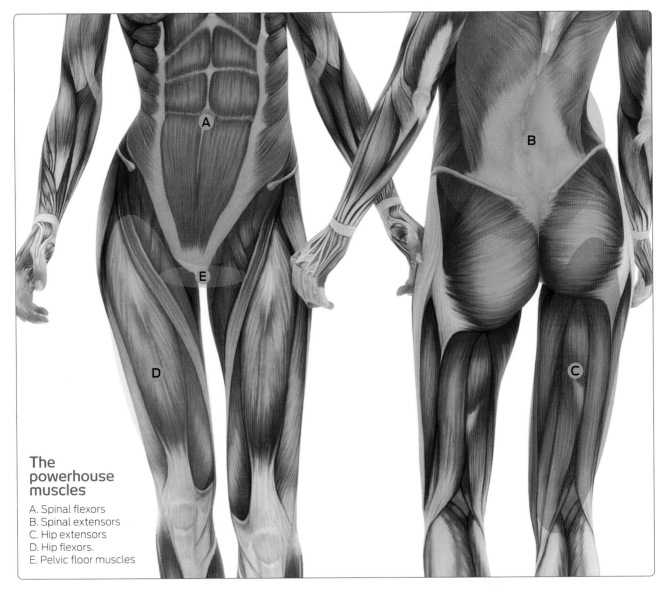

The powerhouse muscles

A. Spinal flexors
B. Spinal extensors
C. Hip extensors
D. Hip flexors.
E. Pelvic floor muscles

Anatomy of the powerhouse

Joseph Pilates never set down in writing the exact components of his conception of the powerhouse, but many Pilates teachers today would broadly define it as the muscles and joints ranging from the pelvic floor to the rib cage, and some would also include the major muscles of the thighs.

The powerhouse muscles can be divided into five major groups: spinal flexors, spinal extensors, hip extensors, hip flexors, and pelvic floor muscles. The components of the group are as follows:

A. Spinal flexors, also known as the anterior abdominals, include the rectus abdominis, transversus abdominis, obliquus internus, and obliquus externus.

B. Spinal extensors, also known as the posterior abdominals, include the erector spinae group (made up of the spinalis, longissimus, and iliocostalis), quadratus lumborum, and multifidus spinae.

C. Hip extensors include the gluteus maximus, gluteus medius, biceps femoris, semitendinosus, semimembranosus, and adductor magnus.

D. Hip flexors include the iliopsoas, sartorius, tensor fasciae latae, pectineus, adductor lingus, gracilis, adductor magnus, rectus femoris, vastus medialis, and vastus lateralis.

E. Pelvic floor muscles include the levator ani, coccygeus, puborectalis, pubococcygeus, and iliococcygeus.

Working the powerhouse

Adhering to the Pilates method can bring about real, positive changes to your body, most noticeably to your posture and to your core. Pilates pays a great deal of attention to

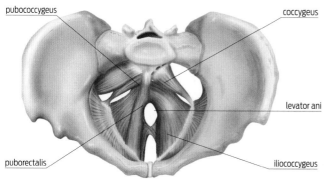

pubococcygeus

coccygeus

levator ani

puborectalis

iliococcygeus

Pelvic floor muscles

Powerhouse joints

Pilates workouts are easy on the joints, making it possible for anyone of any age to take up this low-impact regimen.

The powerhouse joints include the lumbar spinal joints, especially the lumbosacral joint between the lumbar spine and the pelvis, and the hip joints between the pelvis and the thighs.

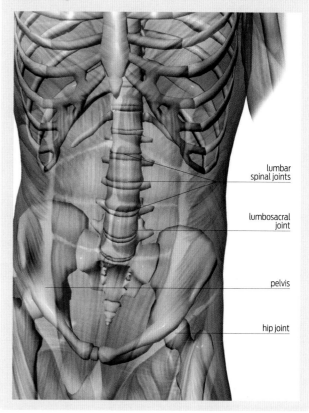

lumbar spinal joints

lumbosacral joint

pelvis

hip joint

pelvic posture, which also determines spinal posture. By concentrating much of its focus on strengthening the girding of muscles that support the pelvis, Pilates truly creates a powerhouse that supports the back.

Pilates exercises also focus on strengthening, stretching, and lengthening your spine. When performing them, think "in and up." This cue will serve as a reminder to straighten your lumbar spine, which also brings your thoracic spine into proper alignment. Better posture helps you look and feel fit—and may help to relieve back problems.

Getting trim

Pilates exercises really work your core, especially the abdominal muscles. By focusing on this crucial area, your core becomes stronger, forming a supportive natural corset for your trunk. A strong, stable core allows you to move with ease and power—and it also gives you a longer, leaner look. And who wouldn't want that?

Pilates at Home

Think of the Pilates method as an ongoing education in body awareness; once you've started your home practice you'll soon feel—and see—how much smarter you're becoming.

We know that the Pilates method trains our body and mind to work together toward a goal of overall fitness and well-being. The goal of the mat work program, at any level, is to create a flow of movement, exercise to exercise, and then to gradually increase the dynamic of the routine while maintaining control of execution. A wonderful quality of the Pilates method is that once you physically and mentally understand its basics, you can carry them out just about anywhere.

Setting up a mat work program

An excellent place to start your study of Pilates is right in your home. It's certainly convenient; home practice can fit into any space or time constraints that you may have.

With mindful practice, you can safely train without an instructor looking over your shoulder, because you'll execute many of the exercises lying on your back in a supine position, lying on your stomach in a prone position, or from a sitting or kneeling start position. Another advantage of practicing at home is that you're not tempted to compare yourself to others in a class, studio, or gym. Instead, you compete with yourself and measure progress against where you've come from—and where you want to go. Yes, this does require self-discipline and motivation. The fact that you're reading these lines in this book, however, means that you're absolutely on the right track. Your exercise routine will soon become one of those indispensable positive habits that will build up your general sense of well-being.

A space of your own

Pilates is a perfect fitness regimen for anyone who likes to work out at home, in private. If you live in a large house or apartment, you may have the luxury of transforming an entire room into a personal Pilates studio, complete with a reformer or other pieces of mega-sized equipment, but even in smaller homes, you can still create a workout area. Basically, your space need not be much larger than your Pilates mat.

Set up your Pilates space away from the clutter of daily life; you want to fully concentrate on the mind-body connection of your exercises without being distracted by clocks, clothes that need folding, or the dog's water bowl that needs refilling. Your space should be clean: you're going to be close to the floor during your entire practice, so it's important that you feel comfortable there. The view of a broom or a vacuum cleaner shouldn't crowd out mental images of your muscles at work. It's also convenient to have a closet or shelf nearby, so that you can store your Pilates equipment and set it up without fuss.

Try to work out in the same place at regular times each week; you want your Pilates practice to become a habit. Creating an inviting sanctuary will further your effort to make it a habit. If simplicity appeals to you, keep your space spare and serene, but don't be afraid to bring in objects that inspire you. A large mirror or anatomical posters of the human skeleton and the major muscles of the back and front might make interesting additions to your space; although not

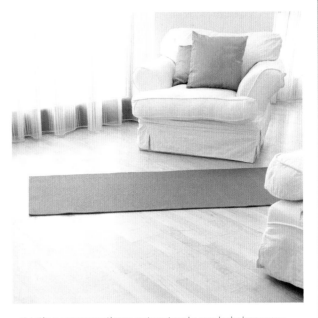

strictly necessary, these extra visuals can help keep you focused while also providing information that can enhance your exercise experience. A vase of fresh flowers may brighten your workout area and your spirits, which may also lift your energy. The more the space appeals to you, the more you will want to go there.

The Pilates mat

Although a folded blanket or towel will serve the purpose, surely the one must-have piece of equipment for just about anyone taking up Pilates is a mat. A mat provides cushioning for your body, especially between your back and the hard floor. Look for a mat that protects your back while still offering support so that you can properly balance and align your body.

Keep in mind that exercise mats are not one-kind-fits-all. A yoga mat, for instance, is thinner that a Pilates mat and slightly sticky so that you can grip the mat during certain poses.

When purchasing a Pilates mat, look for a firm one that is at least one-half inch (1.27 cm) thick. Check its length and width, too. You want one that is long enough for your height and wide enough for you to move easily and fluidly without worrying about shifting off the edges. The roll-up variety typically measures about 72 to 86 inches (180–220 cm), with widths varying from 20 or so inches to close to 40 inches (50–100 cm).

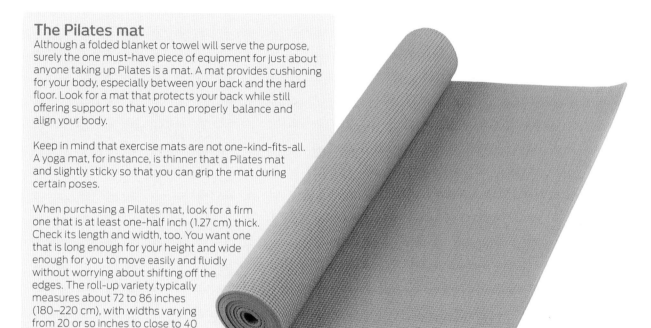

Keep your focus

Go easy on yourself when you begin your practice. At first, the mat work exercises might seem disconnected from your daily activities. Remain patient, and keep your focus on the exercise, on your mental image of the particular anatomical illustration that accompanies each exercise, and on the continuous flow of your breathing. It can be quite difficult to get the essence, the shape, and the breathing all beautifully packaged right from the start.

Exercise add-ons

Once you become comfortable with the basic form of the Pilates exercises, try bringing small pieces of exercise equipment into your home workout. These will make your workout more challenging, allowing you to tailor the exercises to your fitness level as your ability improves with time and practice. Crucially, these pieces of equipment can also lend variety to your fitness regimen.

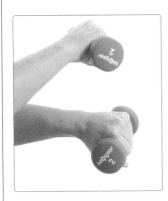

Hand weights can be incorporated into Pilates exercises to enhance strengthening and toning benefits—making an exercise that little bit more challenging.

The Pilates ball, a small inflatable ball, usually measuring about 9 inches (23 cm) in diameter, serves multiple purposes.

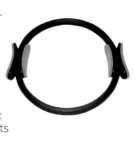

Grasp it between your knees to engage the hard-to-tone muscles of the inner thighs or place it behind your back to lend extra support during mat work. Any small, soft ball can achieve this effect. A foam roller also provides cushioning. Available in a variety of sizes, materials, and densities, you can also use it for stretching, strengthening, balance training, stability training, and self-massage.

You can also look for other Pilates-specific equipment, such as the fitness circle. Also known as a magic circle, it is a flexible ring, usually made of metal, with pliable handles that adds resistance to a Pilates movement when you squeeze its sides together.

Learning new exercises is similar to learning new words in a foreign language. The sounds, structure, and meaning only become clear over time—and with practice. And it's only after you've picked up some vocabulary that you can begin to construct sentences (exercise sequences) and connect these sentences to form cohesive and fluid paragraphs (your exercise regimen). Remember, too, that no matter how many times you've performed the exercises in your fitness routine, there'll still be new elements and subtleties to discover, new layers of exploration to savor, and old images to spark your imagination and become useful with renewed force.

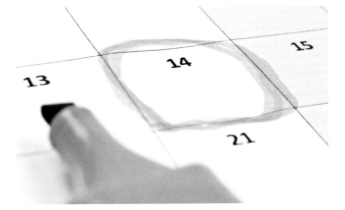

Making time for Pilates

Joseph Pilates suggested that anyone practicing Pilates should start out attempting a few of the exercises in sequential order for just 10 minutes a day, four days a week, for at least three months. His belief—which still rings true today—was that the positive results of your workout session should motivate you to increase the number of exercises you perform in subsequent sessions. This makes sense: the obvious rewards and benefits of the Pilates method will increase your desire to do more—and do it more often.

Set a realistic goal for yourself. Ten minutes a day for four days a week would be good; 20 minutes a day for two days a week would also be good. Stay realistic and commit to following your training schedule for three months, as Joseph Pilates suggested. After this period, you'll have enough perspective to reevaluate your training, your scheduling, and your level of skill, and then establish a new set of goals for the next three-month period.

Life happens, as the truism goes. If there are days when you can't roll out your mat and occupy your private exercise space for whatever reason, remember: it's okay! Do a 10-minute exercise variation while stuck in traffic, holding onto an overhead pole in a rush-hour subway, or standing on a checkout line at the supermarket. Bring your Pilates training into your daily round of diverse activities.

Equipment

You actually have everything you need to start practicing Pilates right now, today. You have your body, your intelligence, and your ability to use mindful images to affect your movement patterns. That's quite a lot already, isn't it?

Joseph Pilates believed that his exercises could be performed either on the floor or on a mat. Nowadays, a so-called Pilates mat is considered to be an exercise essential because of the support and comfort it provides. Pilates mats are usually affordable and available in a variety of places, from mega sports stores to large bookstores, as well as online. If no mat is at hand, you can work directly on the (clean) floor, or use a blanket or towel to soften your contact with the hard surface.

Small pieces of equipment such as exercise balls, resistance bands, small hand weights, fitness circles, or foam rollers can all add variety and challenge to your home training.

What to wear

Any comfortable exercise clothes that allow you full range of motion are fine for your Pilates workout sessions. Avoid too much free-flowing fabric; it can easily get in the way of your movements. Pick close-fitting tops and bottoms streamlined to your body shape so that you don't have to fidget and readjust your clothes after every movement.

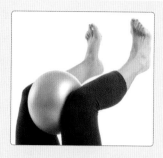

Using a Pilates ball

Several of the exercises in this book feature the Pilates ball, and many others show its use in a modification or advanced version. In the classic exercise the Hundred (see pages 28–31), the ball serves as a physical reminder that your legs should always be dynamically active and strongly held together, even though the main action of the exercise may seem to be happening in your arms, which are moving rapidly and strongly up and down. Using the ball helps you to grasp the shape and dynamic of an exercise.

Remember—you shouldn't blow a Pilates ball up all the way; instead, there should be a little give on the surface.

Like yoga, Pilates is best performed barefoot, so that you get the most traction possible. To protect your feet from exposure to foot fungi and other germs, which may occur in commercial fitness centers and studios in which numerous people use the same equipment, look for specially made Pilates socks or slippers. These are lightweight with slip-free soles. They'll also keep you firmly grounded if your feet tend to sweat during physical exertion.

How to use this book

Begin with "Best of the Classics," and practice just a few exercises at a time until you feel confident in your ability to perform them. For all of the exercises, you'll find a short overview of the move, photos with step-by-step instructions demonstrating how to do it, some tips on how to perform it, and anatomical illustrations that highlight key muscles. Some exercises have accompanying variations, shown in the modification box.

Alongside each exercise is a quick-read panel that features an at-a-glance illustration of the targeted areas, an estimate of the level of difficulty, and the average amount of time you'll need to complete the exercise. The last category is a caution list: if you have one of the issues listed, it is best to avoid that exercise.

This information is here for you, but don't feel pressured to use it all at once. You should focus on the kind of information (visual or textual, for example) that best suits your learning style. There will always be things that you miss the first time around, so come back periodically to leaf through these pages in order to check up on your form and understanding of the exercises.

Pilates and Nutrition

Eating a balanced, healthy diet is essential. Focus on fresh, high-quality foods that boost energy without adding toxins to your body.

The connection between fitness and nutrition has long been emphasized, and for good reason. Whether you are taking up Pilates to get it shape or to improve the shape you're in, eating the proper quantity and balance of nutrients is essential to achieving your goals. Consuming the right types and amounts of nutrients and fluid helps you to exercise for longer periods and at a higher intensity. It also aids in muscle recovery after workouts, improves strength, increases energy levels, helps to maintain healthy immune function, and reduces the risk of injury and heat cramps.

Fueling for fitness

Our bodies need fuel to function, and the harder we push ourselves the more fuel we require. Professional athletes and marathon runners utilize carbohydrate loading and require hundreds of excess calories to keep them performing at their peak. But for most of us, who work out less than four times a week at low to moderate intensity, it is not necessary to take these drastic measures. Instead, as you begin practicing Pilates, focus on consuming small meals with plenty of fruits, vegetables, whole grains, and nuts. Look to take in a healthy combination of carbohydrates and protein with small amounts of fat and fiber. For example, try eating a nut butter sandwich on whole-wheat toast with an apple or a serving of Greek yogurt with fruit and low-fat granola approximately three to four hours before exercising. Then, about one half hour to an hour before working out, eat a whole fruit like a banana or orange and drink a full glass of water. The proper timing and intake of these nutrients will enhance your workout and the benefits you receive from it.

After a workout, carbohydrates help to replenish muscle fuel lost during exercise, while protein aids in the repair of damaged muscle tissue and the development of new tissue. Aim to eat a meal or snack 15 to 60 minutes after engaging in physical activity. Some healthful meal suggestions include a chicken or vegetable stir-fry, whole-wheat pita with turkey, hummus, and salad, or a brown rice bowl with beans and steamed vegetables. If you are on the go and cannot prepare a healthful meal within the hour, stock your gym bag with nutritional supplements. A variety of bars on the market contain a balanced blend of carbohydrates, protein, and essential vitamins and minerals.

A little protein goes a long way

There is a common misconception that loading up on protein is the key to building muscle mass. Although protein plays an important role in the growth and repair of muscle tissue, most adults who live in developed countries already get more than enough from their typical daily diets.

For adults engaging in approximately one hour of exercise three (or fewer) times a week, the daily recommendation for protein is 46 grams for women and 56 grams for men. One ounce of meat, poultry, or fish, which is similar in size to a small matchbox, contains 7 grams of protein. This means that 6.5 ounces of meat, fish, or poultry provides the average woman with all the protein she needs in a day, and 8 ounces meets the daily protein requirement for most men. The portion of protein provided by one main dish at many restaurants comes close to meeting these needs all on its own! Many individuals, especially those who dine

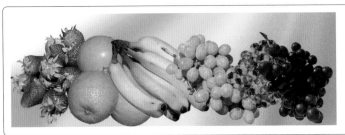

A rainbow diet

Eating the colors of the rainbow may sound like an elementary school lesson plan, but its underlying message is important for adults and children alike. Choose from a varied palette of fruits and vegetables from red berries to green spinach to violet plums—and all the shades in between. Splashing your plate with different-colored fruits and vegetables is an easy and smart way to ensure that you are getting the vitamins and minerals you need.

out frequently, are exceeding their protein needs by more than just a few grams. In many cases, men with moderate-intensity workout regimens consume the same amount of protein that professional athletes consume. Exceeding the recommended amount of protein is unnecessary and can even prove harmful.

Popular animal proteins like eggs, beef, and pork are packed with saturated fat and cholesterol. An abundance of medium- and high-fat animal proteins in the diet increases risk of heart disease and can also place unwarranted burden on the kidneys. Too often, those of us who eat high-fat diets don't get enough of other kinds of food. These diets are typically lacking in fruits and vegetables, leading to an insufficient intake of important nutrients like vitamin C, vitamin E, and folate. The bottom line is that you are most likely getting enough protein in your diet, but you may be getting it from the wrong foods. Choose smarter sources of protein such as tuna, salmon, chicken, turkey, nuts, and beans, and complement them with a variety of fruits and vegetables. This will help you to achieve your physical fitness goals while also increasing your energy levels and keep your heart and internal organs healthier.

Eat your veggies

What's not to like about vegetables? They are generally low-fat, low-calorie foods with a high return in vitamins and minerals— especially the green, yellow, and orange ones, which are great sources of calcium, magnesium, potassium, iron, beta-carotene, vitamin B complex, vitamin C, vitamin A, and vitamin K. As an added benefit, most vegetables contain soluble and insoluble dietary fiber.

Aim to include about 5 to 7 servings of fresh vegetables in your daily diet. Look for seasonal varieties in a rich array of colors. Look for fresh, whole vegetables that are bright in color and feel heavy for their sizes. Whenever possible, buy small quantities that you can consume in just a day or two.

Getting your vitamins

Vitamins C and E as well as iron are recognized as especially beneficial to physically active people. Each of these nutrients contains unique properties that contribute to aerobic endurance, immune system strength, and optimal recovery from exercise. Nuts, seeds, and plant oils like sunflower oil are great sources of vitamin E, while citrus fruits, blueberries, strawberries, red peppers, and broccoli supply vitamin C. Spinach, kidney beans, and fortified grain products, such as breakfast cereals, contain iron, but our bodies are less able to absorb it from these foods than from animal sources such as meat and seafood.

Hydrate, hydrate

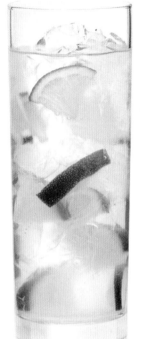

Consuming adequate fluid is another key factor in maximizing exercise performance and preventing injury. Proper hydration maintains optimal organ function and helps you feel your best during and after your Pilates practice. It is healthy to work up a sweat while exercising; sweating is your body's way of protecting you from overheating during periods of physical exertion. When you fail to replace fluids lost through perspiration, serious issues can present. Early signs of dehydration include thirst, flushed skin, premature fatigue, increased pulse rate and breathing, and decreased exercise capacity. These symptoms can give way to dizziness and severe weakness if dehydration is allowed to persist. Most nutrition authorities recommend drinking water before, during, and after low- to moderate-intensity exercise that lasts up to an hour. For anyone exercising for more than an hour at a higher intensity, it is beneficial to consume beverages that contain a combination of carbohydrates and electrolytes. A smart choice is 100 percent pure coconut

water, which contains fewer calories and less sugar and sodium than many popular sports drinks. Another healthy way to replace fluids and electrolytes lost during exercise is to eat a serving of fruit or vegetables after your workout.

Control your body's destiny

Maintaining a healthy diet requires the right mind-set and a sufficient dose of determination. Life happens: we get invited to parties, suffer stressful days, and succumb to the occasional overwhelming chocolate craving. Nobody said that it was going to be as simple as waving a magic wand and never wanting French fries again! If you initiate a healthier diet by making drastic changes, it is unlikely to last; eating lettuce and broccoli for lunch and dinner Monday through Friday and then topping off a pint of chocolate fudge ice cream every weekend on "cheat days" is an inefficient and unhealthy approach to meeting your health and weight-loss goals. Starting with smart, measurable goals and staying on a realistic and positive path is the best way to achieve long-term results.

Find a balance that works for you. Make sure that your daily diet includes foods you enjoy so that you do not enter the weekend feeling deprived. Find healthier substitutes for the less healthful foods you crave. Want chocolate? Some nutritional supplement bars deliver rich chocolate flavor to your taste buds while also providing you with 100 percent of the daily-recommended folate. They may even satisfy your sweet tooth equally well as your favorite candy bar (which contains three times the saturated fat)!

Leading a healthier lifestyle need not mean forfeiting your social life. Dining out with friends and attending dinner parties may present more of a challenge than before, but with the right navigation tools they can be just as enjoyable. The number one rule: never arrive at a restaurant or party

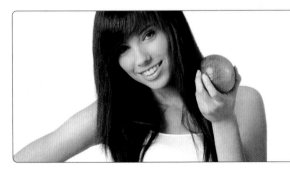

Exercising and energy

Should you take a bite of that apple? We're all quite different as human beings, and some of us feel that we have to eat something before our Pilates session so that our exercising isn't accompanied by stomach grumbles and dizziness. Others of us work better with little in our stomachs. Whatever works for you is—most probably—good for you. Your goal is to have the energy to carry out an intense, dynamic, and invigorating fitness workout, so make sure that you have enough nourishment for your body and mind to work in harmony—creating and maintaining a happy, vitalized, and healthy you.

Vitamins and supplements

It is always best to obtain nutrients from whole foods. If you find certain nutrient-rich foods unpalatable or they aren't readily available where you live, however, then it is crucial to take a multivitamin that contains at least 100 percent of the recommended daily value (DV) for the nutrients you need. This information can be found on the supplement package.

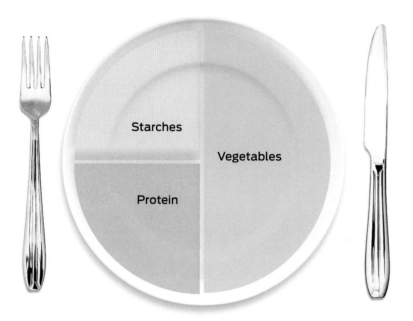

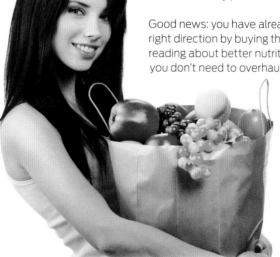

everyone at the table wants to share—a great way to ensure portion control while still enjoying a sweet ending to the night.

At a dinner party, serve yourself instead of letting other people dictate what goes on your plate. When you look at your blank plate, imagine it as a diagram cut into three sections. Designate the upper left corner for starches like pasta and rice, the lower left corner for protein like turkey, chicken, or fish and the entire right side of the plate for vegetables. This will help you to retain portion control and consume a balanced meal.

Do not eat quickly: scientific research has shown that it takes 20 minutes for your brain to process whether or not your stomach is full. Savor each bite and chew thoroughly to allow your brain to catch up to the state of your stomach. Once you have licked the last crumb off your plate, place your hands in your lap and make a conscious decision not to go back for seconds—at least not yet. Occupy your mind and mouth for 20 minutes by talking to friends, helping the host clear the table, or even visiting the bathroom and reciting a monologue in front of the mirror if need be! Once the 20 minutes are up you will have a better grasp on your level of satiation. If you are still hungry, go back for the vegetable choices and drink another glass of water. Use your willpower to avoid second helpings of starch and fatty proteins like beef or pork.

too hungry. Eat a whole fruit like an apple or orange and drink two glasses of water one half hour before mealtime. If you are in a rush, have your fruit and water en route to your destination. This small healthy snack will help you make better decisions and forgo nutritionally scanty starters like bread or chips and dip.

When dining out, order a healthy starter when you get to the table so that you are less tempted to pick at the contents of the bread basket. If possible, review the restaurant's offerings online beforehand to reduce the stress of finding healthy dishes on the spot. Do not be timid about asking your server to describe the contents of a sauce or how a main dish is prepared. She is there to help you and your desire to eat healthfully is something to be proud of. Avoid fried foods and cream-based sauces such as Alfredo or vodka sauce. Instead, opt for dishes made with light olive oil or marinara sauce. If you are really craving something sweet at the end of your meal, order a dessert that

Good news: you have already taken a step in the right direction by buying this fitness book and reading about better nutrition. More good news: you don't need to overhaul your life or refrigerator to achieve your goals. Initiating small changes, like substituting healthier choices for the less nutritious foods in your diet, can get you looking and feeling better as you move through your daily life.

Full-body Anatomy

Front view
Annotation Key
* indicates deep muscles

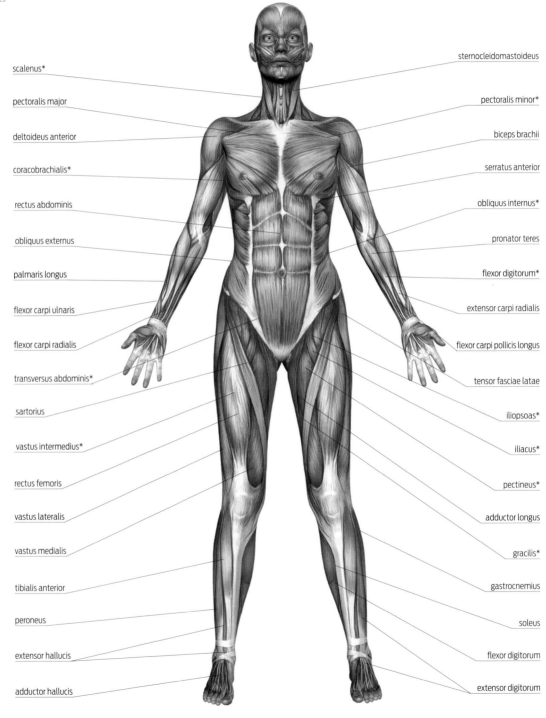

scalenus*

pectoralis major

deltoideus anterior

coracobrachialis*

rectus abdominis

obliquus externus

palmaris longus

flexor carpi ulnaris

flexor carpi radialis

transversus abdominis*

sartorius

vastus intermedius*

rectus femoris

vastus lateralis

vastus medialis

tibialis anterior

peroneus

extensor hallucis

adductor hallucis

sternocleidomastoideus

pectoralis minor*

biceps brachii

serratus anterior

obliquus internus*

pronator teres

flexor digitorum*

extensor carpi radialis

flexor carpi pollicis longus

tensor fasciae latae

iliopsoas*

iliacus*

pectineus*

adductor longus

gracilis*

gastrocnemius

soleus

flexor digitorum

extensor digitorum

Back view
Annotation Key
* indicates deep muscles

semispinalis*

trapezius

deltoideus
medialis

infraspinatus*

deltoideus posterior

teres minor

subscapularis*

triceps brachii

rhomboideus*

anconeus

multifidus spinae*

gemellus superior*

quadratus femoris*

obturator internus*

obturator externus

vastus lateralis

gemellus inferior*

adductor magnus

plantaris

gastrocnemius

soleus

flexor digitorum

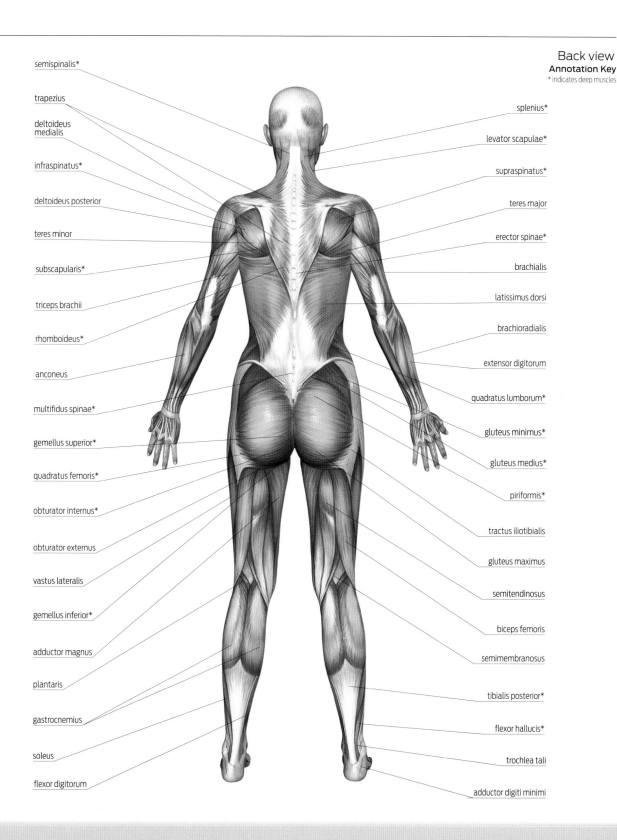

splenius*

levator scapulae*

supraspinatus*

teres major

erector spinae*

brachialis

latissimus dorsi

brachioradialis

extensor digitorum

quadratus lumborum*

gluteus minimus*

gluteus medius*

piriformis*

tractus iliotibialis

gluteus maximus

semitendinosus

biceps femoris

semimembranosus

tibialis posterior*

flexor hallucis*

trochlea tali

adductor digiti minimi

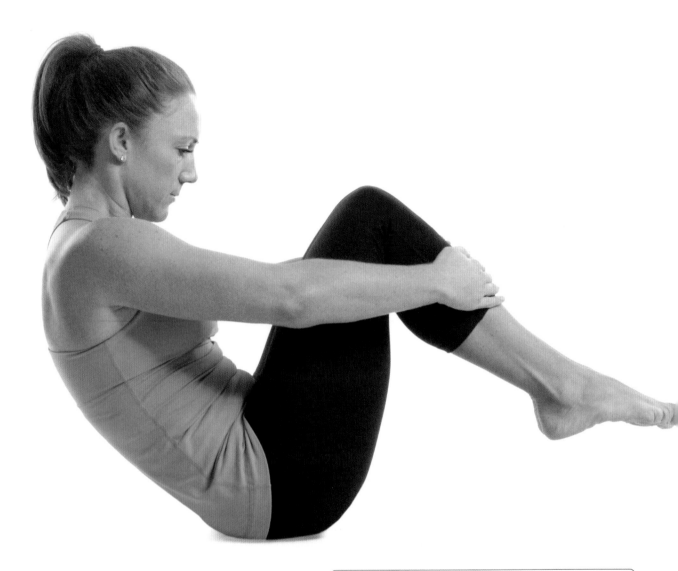

Contents

According to Joseph Pilates, "physical fitness is the first requisite of happiness," and he made it his life's mission to design a fitness regimen that addresses both mind and body. For nearly 40 years, Pilates taught his ground-breaking method, and a group of his students later continued his legacy, committing themselves to passing along his work just as he had taught it.

This method has since been labeled classical Pilates, and it features at its core the group of exercises first devised by Pilates himself. The following is a sampling some of the best of the classics.

Best of the Classics

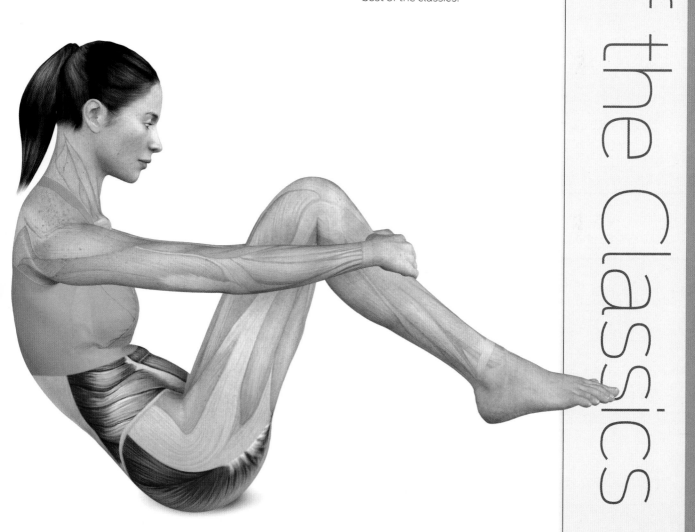

Hundred I

The first of the classical Pilates exercises, Hundred I is effective for warming up the body. It's a breathing exercise that focuses your awareness on the area of your core stability— that powerhouse that consists of the abdominals, buttocks, lower back, and hips.

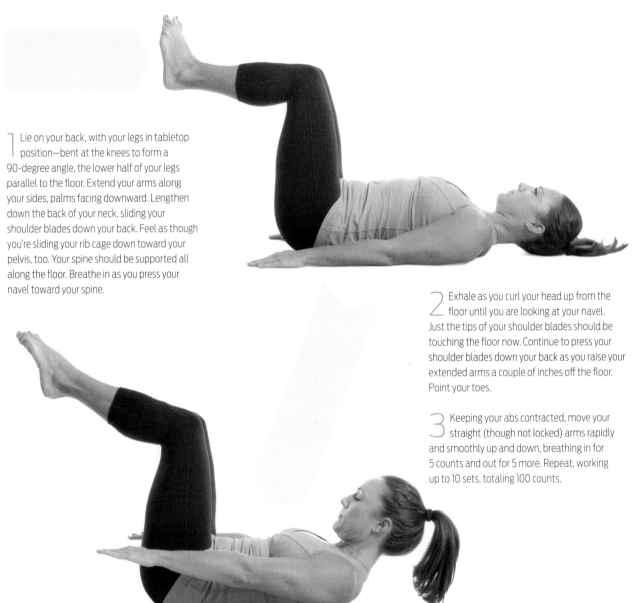

1 Lie on your back, with your legs in tabletop position—bent at the knees to form a 90-degree angle, the lower half of your legs parallel to the floor. Extend your arms along your sides, palms facing downward. Lengthen down the back of your neck, sliding your shoulder blades down your back. Feel as though you're sliding your rib cage down toward your pelvis, too. Your spine should be supported all along the floor. Breathe in as you press your navel toward your spine.

2 Exhale as you curl your head up from the floor until you are looking at your navel. Just the tips of your shoulder blades should be touching the floor now. Continue to press your shoulder blades down your back as you raise your extended arms a couple of inches off the floor. Point your toes.

3 Keeping your abs contracted, move your straight (though not locked) arms rapidly and smoothly up and down, breathing in for 5 counts and out for 5 more. Repeat, working up to 10 sets, totaling 100 counts.

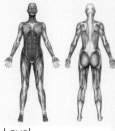

Correct form
· Keep the back of your neck long and the front of your neck open.
· Press your shoulder blades down your back.
· Imagine an orange under your chin as you curl your head upward.
· Actively engage the muscles of your abdominals, buttocks, and legs.
· Keep your torso and legs stabilized.

Avoid
· "Popping" your abdominal muscles outward.
· Tensing the muscles in your neck.
· Allowing your shoulders to roll forward.
· Moving your upper body or legs during the exercise.

Annotation Key
Bold text indicates target muscles
Black text indicates other working muscles
* indicates deep muscles

Level
· Beginner

Duration
· 2–3 minutes

Benefits
· Strengthens and stabilizes core muscles
· Increases blood circulation
· Supports optimal breathing patterns

Caution
· History of cervical spine injury
· Neck pain or stiffness

rectus abdominis

pectoralis major

vastus lateralis

rectus femoris

vastus intermedius*

transversus abdominis*

tensor fasciae latae

obliquus internus*

obliquus externus

deltoideus anterior

triceps brachii

teres major

Front View

iliopsoas *
pectineus*
adductor magnus
sartorius
adductor longus
gracilis*
vastus medialis

Modifications
Harder: To add extra lower-body resistance and awareness, perform the exercise with a Pilates ball between your legs.

Hundred II

Hundred II is an advanced version of Hundred I. Attempt this version only after you begin to feel comfortable and confident with the basic exercise. Hundred II calls for you to work with your legs extended off the mat, which requires much more control of your core muscles. Your spinal imprint should remain constant throughout the exercise, too.

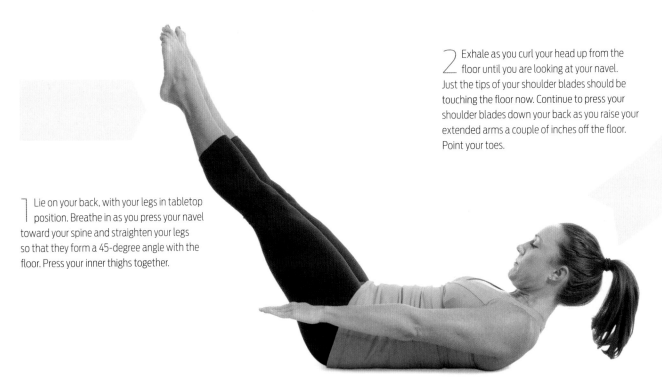

2 Exhale as you curl your head up from the floor until you are looking at your navel. Just the tips of your shoulder blades should be touching the floor now. Continue to press your shoulder blades down your back as you raise your extended arms a couple of inches off the floor. Point your toes.

1 Lie on your back, with your legs in tabletop position. Breathe in as you press your navel toward your spine and straighten your legs so that they form a 45-degree angle with the floor. Press your inner thighs together.

Correct form
· Keep the back of your neck long and your throat open.
· Hold your legs together as if they were a single leg.
· Keep your legs extended at a 45-degree angle from the floor.
· Press your shoulder blades down your back.
· Keep your arms and legs strong, though not stiff.
· Keep your coccyx firmly planted into the floor.
· Engage the muscles of your abdominals, buttocks, and legs.
· Keep your torso and legs stabilized.
· Keep your chest open.

Avoid
· Holding your breath.
· Letting your head bob up and down along with your arms.
· Lifting your shoulders.
· Locking your knees.
· "Popping" your abdominal muscles outward.
· Tensing the muscles in your neck.

Modifications
Harder: Perform the exercise while holding a Pilates ball between your knees or ankles.

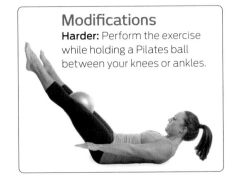

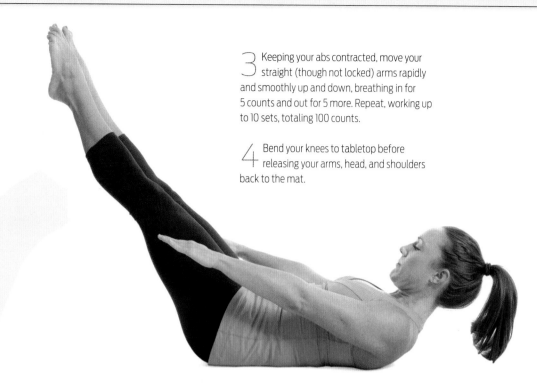

3 Keeping your abs contracted, move your straight (though not locked) arms rapidly and smoothly up and down, breathing in for 5 counts and out for 5 more. Repeat, working up to 10 sets, totaling 100 counts.

4 Bend your knees to tabletop before releasing your arms, head, and shoulders back to the mat.

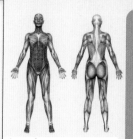

Level
· Advanced

Duration

· 2–4 minutes

Benefits
· Strengthens and stabilizes core muscles
· Strengthens legs
· Supports optimal breathing patterns

Caution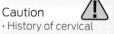
· History of cervical spine injury
· Knee injury
· Neck pain or stiffness

Annotation Key
Bold text indicates target muscles
Black text indicates other working muscles
* indicates deep muscles

Front View

iliopsoas *

pectineus*
adductor magnus
adductor longus
sartorius
gracilis*
vastus medialis

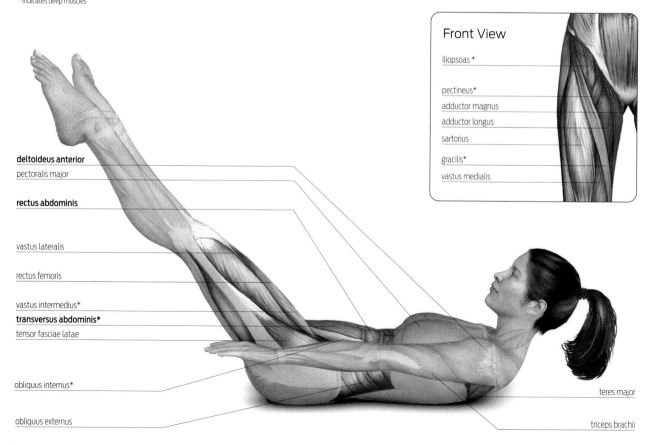

deltoideus anterior
pectoralis major

rectus abdominis

vastus lateralis

rectus femoris

vastus intermedius*
transversus abdominis*
tensor fasciae latae

obliquus internus*

obliquus externus

teres major

triceps brachii

Roll-Up

The classical Pilates Roll-Up will challenge your powerhouse muscles, flatten your abdominals, and strengthen your back. Let your breath guide you through the exercise, so that you use the same control rolling down as you do rolling up. Master this one and your abdominals and back will thank you.

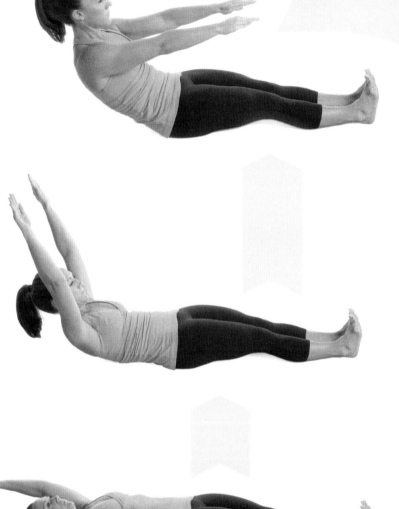

1 Lie on your back, with your spine in neutral position and your ankles strongly flexed. Glide your shoulder blades down your back as you lift your arms overhead, extended slightly above the mat behind you. Press your shoulders and your rib cage downward.

2 Press your navel to your spine, and, in sequence, roll up each vertebra from the mat, reaching your arms forward into the space above your legs. It helps to really press your heels into the mat.

3 Reverse the movement, rolling back down to the mat vertebra by vertebra, resisting the urge to lift your shoulders and collapse your chest.

4 Complete 5 repetitions.

Correct form
· Keep your abdominals and rib cage strongly interlaced with your back.
· Keep pressing your legs and heels into the mat for stabilization.

Avoid
· Using shoulder or arm momentum to roll up or down.
· Bouncing or otherwise compromising the fluid steadiness of the movements.

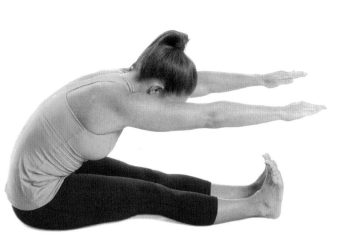

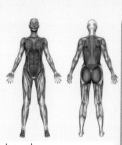

Level
· Intermediate

Duration
· 2–3 minutes

Benefits
· Challenges core muscles
· Tightens abdominals
· Strengthens back
· Mobilizes spine

Caution
· Herniated disc

Annotation Key
Bold text indicates target muscles
Black text indicates other working muscles
* indicates deep muscles

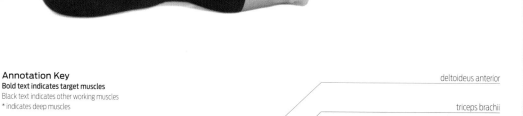

deltoideus anterior

triceps brachii

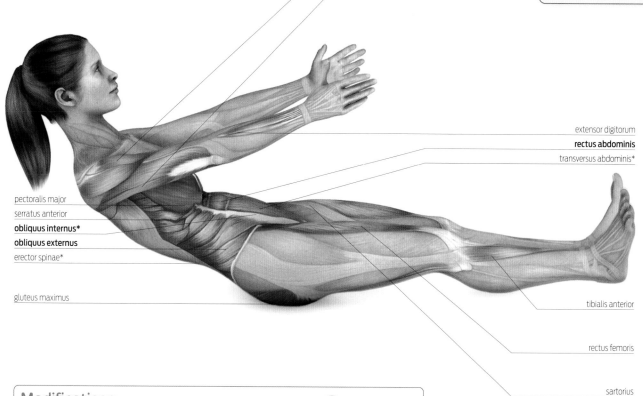

extensor digitorum
rectus abdominis
transversus abdominis*

pectoralis major
serratus anterior
obliquus internus*
obliquus externus
erector spinae*

gluteus maximus

tibialis anterior

rectus femoris

sartorius

Modifications
Harder: Grasp a Pilates ball as you perform the exercise. Keep your arms extended and the ball stable throughout the exercise.

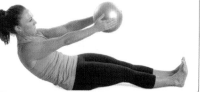

Rollover

Another Pilates exercise from the original canon, Rollover stretches and articulates your spine. It requires a high degree of core control and awareness.

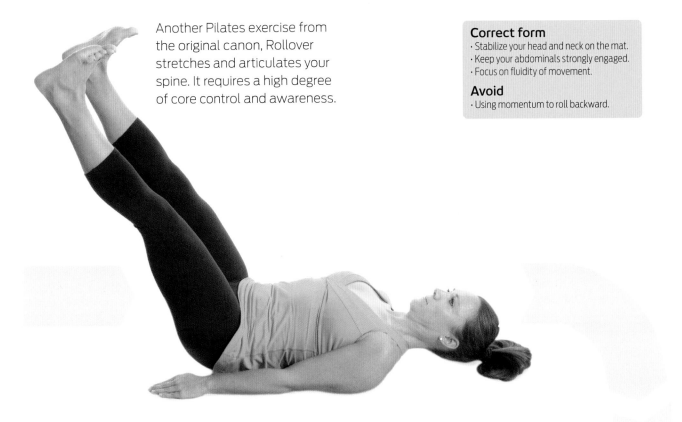

1 Lie on your back with your arms along your sides, palms down.

2 Lift your legs so that they form a 45-degree angle with the mat, and flex your ankles. Engage your abdominals, and make sure that your spine is stable on the mat.

3 Press your arms into the mat to help stabilize your torso and roll your extended legs back toward your head, carefully peeling your spine off the mat.

4 When you have reached the farthest position, open your leg slightly. With control, roll sequentially through your spine to return your legs to the starting position above your hips.

5 Complete 4 to 6 repetitions.

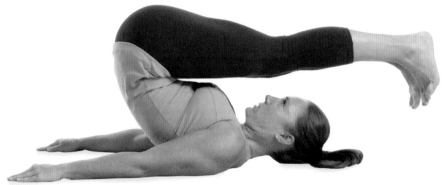

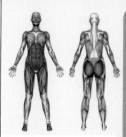

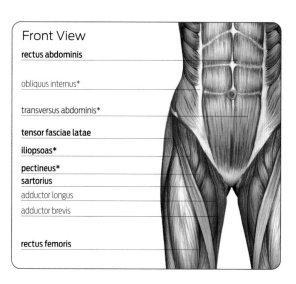

Front View

rectus abdominis

obliquus internus*

transversus abdominis*

tensor fasciae latae

iliopsoas*

pectineus*

sartorius

adductor longus

adductor brevis

rectus femoris

Annotation Key
Bold text indicates target muscles
Black text indicates other working muscles
* indicates deep muscles

Level
· Intermediate

Duration
· 2–3 minutes

Benefits
· Stretches and
  mobilizes spine
· Challenges core

Caution
· Cervical spine issues
· Herniated disc

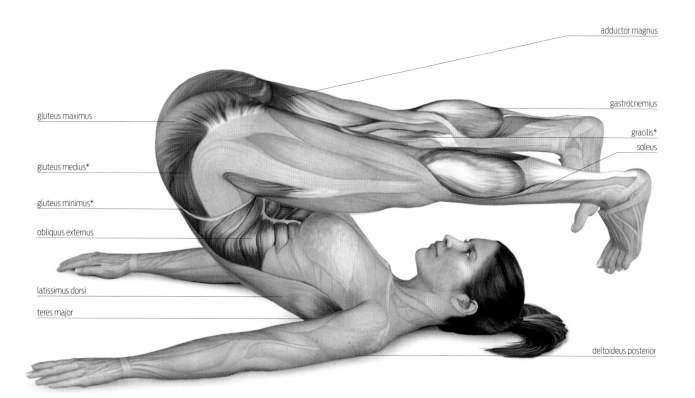

adductor magnus

gluteus maximus

gastrocnemius

gracilis*

soleus

gluteus medius*

gluteus minimus*

obliquus externus

latissimus dorsi

teres major

deltoideus posterior

One-Leg Circle

One-Leg Circle develops stability of the
lumbar spine and pelvis, while increasing
mobility in your hip joints and strengthening
your anterior leg muscles. It improves your
ability to initiate the movement of your leg
from deep in your hip socket, independently
of your pelvis.

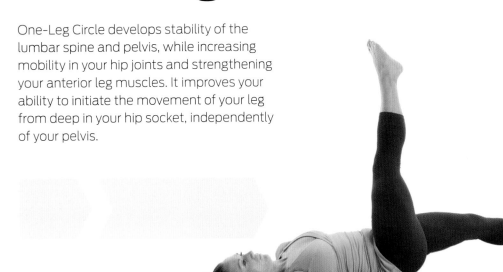

1 Lie on your back with a neutral pelvis,
your legs bent and parallel, feet planted into
your mat and knees aligned with your hip bones.
Your arms should be long by your sides, shoulder
blades stabilized.

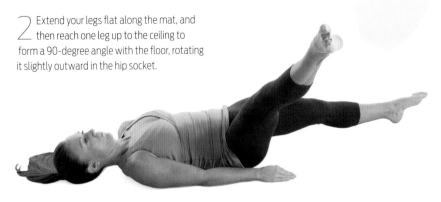

2 Extend your legs flat along the mat, and
then reach one leg up to the ceiling to
form a 90-degree angle with the floor, rotating
it slightly outward in the hip socket.

3 From your hip socket, "draw" small circles
with your leg: inhale for the first half of
each circle as the leg crosses the midline of your
body and then downward, and exhale for the
second half as you move your leg sideward and
up to the starting position again. Pause briefly
at the top of each circle as a marker of control
and completion.

4 Circle 5 times in one direction and then
5 times in the other direction. Switch legs,
and repeat.

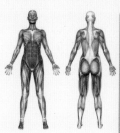

Back View

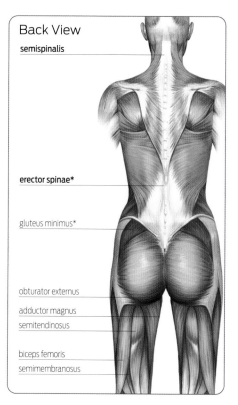

semispinalis

erector spinae*

gluteus minimus*

obturator externus

adductor magnus

semitendinosus

biceps femoris

semimembranosus

Front View

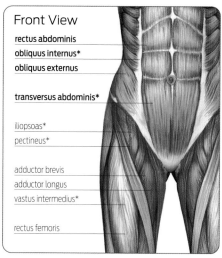

rectus abdominis

obliquus internus*

obliquus externus

transversus abdominis*

iliopsoas*

pectineus*

adductor brevis

adductor longus

vastus intermedius*

rectus femoris

Annotation Key
Bold text indicates target muscles
Black text indicates other working muscles
* indicates deep muscles

Level
· Beginner/
  Intermediate

Duration
· 2–4 minutes

Benefits
· Articulates,
  stretches, and
  strengthens leg
  in hip socket

Caution
· Lower-back issues

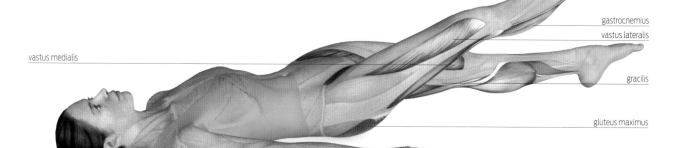

vastus medialis

soleus

gastrocnemius

vastus lateralis

gracilis

gluteus maximus

Modifications

Easier: Perform the exercise with one leg bent, with the foot flat on the floor as your other leg circles.

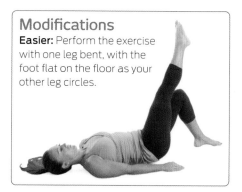

Correct form

· Keep your rib cage and shoulder blades stabilized throughout the exercise.
· Keep your pelvis level at all times.
· Think of engaging your buttocks to perform the movement.
· Make the circles small and fluid so that pelvic stability is never compromised.
· Keep the knee of your bottom leg straight and the whole leg engaged throughout the exercise.

Avoid

· Straining your neck or shoulders.
· Losing control of your neutral pelvis.
· Creating any movement in your lumbar spine.

Rolling Like a Ball

Rolling Like a Ball is one of the very few Pilates exercises that use momentum. The rolling dynamic works your abdominals, improves your sense of balance, and supports the flexibility of your spine. At the same time, this exercise challenges your ability to continually control your abdominals while rolling back and forth.

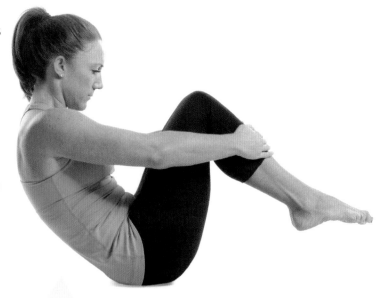

1 Balance at the front edge of your mat with your slightly turned-out knees tucked in toward your chest, your feet close to your buttocks, and your weight just behind your sit-bones. Place your hands on your shins, press your shoulders down your back, and hold your elbows slightly away from your body.

2 In this c-curve form, with abdominals pressing toward your spine, inhale, and roll backward.

3 Scoop your abdominals even more as you exhale, which will supply the momentum for you to roll forward to balance again.

4 Repeat 4 to 6 times.

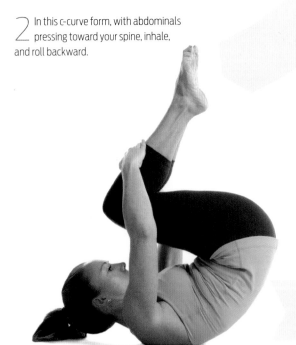

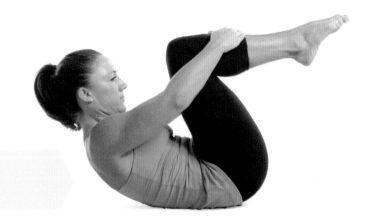

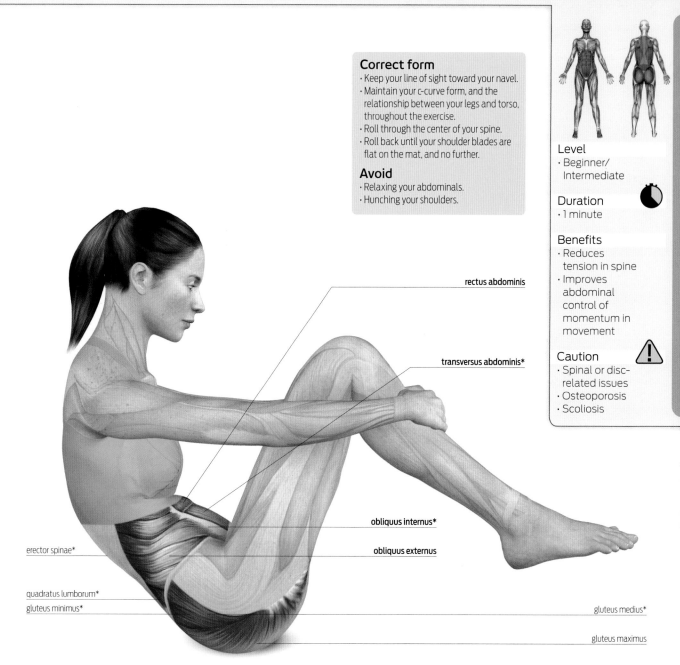

Correct form
· Keep your line of sight toward your navel.
· Maintain your c-curve form, and the relationship between your legs and torso, throughout the exercise.
· Roll through the center of your spine.
· Roll back until your shoulder blades are flat on the mat, and no further.

Avoid
· Relaxing your abdominals.
· Hunching your shoulders.

Level
· Beginner/ Intermediate

Duration
· 1 minute

Benefits
· Reduces tension in spine
· Improves abdominal control of momentum in movement

Caution
· Spinal or disc-related issues
· Osteoporosis
· Scoliosis

rectus abdominis

transversus abdominis*

obliquus internus*

obliquus externus

erector spinae*

quadratus lumborum*

gluteus minimus*

gluteus medius*

gluteus maximus

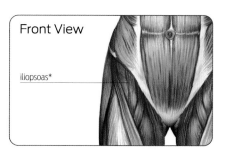

Front View

iliopsoas*

Annotation Key
Bold text indicates target muscles
Black text indicates other working muscles
* indicates deep muscles

Single-Leg Stretch

Single-Leg Stretch—the first of a group called the "stomach series"—improves your core stability while your arms and legs are moving (quickly). This exercise requires coordination, as well as control of your deep abdominal muscles. It's important to think of your powerhouse and precise positions as you perform this exercise, so that your legs and torso don't begin to tip and tilt like a rowboat in a storm at sea.

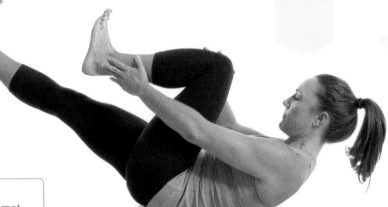

1 Lie on your back with your legs in tabletop position, your spine extended along the floor and your knees bent so that your legs form a 90-degree angle, feet flexed. Your neck should be long, your throat open, your shoulder blades stabilized, and your arms extended along your sides, palms down.

2 To prepare, inhale while curling the top of your head forward so that you are looking between your knees. Place your hands on the outsides of your calves.

Modifications
Easier: Keep your head on the mat throughout the exercise.

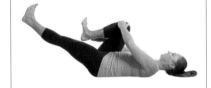

3 Exhale, and extend one leg diagonally to form a 45-degree angle with the floor, bringing your outside hand to your ankle and your inside hand to your knee.

4 Inhale, and begin to switch hands and legs.

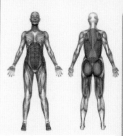

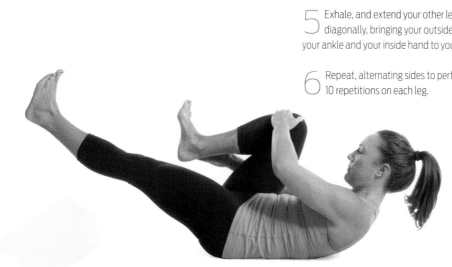

5 Exhale, and extend your other leg diagonally, bringing your outside hand to your ankle and your inside hand to your knee.

6 Repeat, alternating sides to perform 6 to 10 repetitions on each leg.

Level
· Beginner/ Intermediate

Duration

· 2–3 minutes

Benefits
· Strengthens and stabilizes core

Caution

· Cervical spine issues
· Neck strain

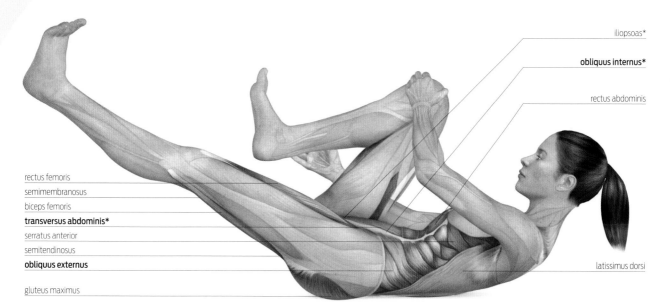

iliopsoas*

obliquus internus*

rectus abdominis

rectus femoris

semimembranosus

biceps femoris

transversus abdominis*

serratus anterior

semitendinosus

obliquus externus

gluteus maximus

latissimus dorsi

Correct form
· Engage your buttocks to maximize control over your legs.
· Keep your neck long and your shoulder blades pressed downward, away from your ears.

Avoid
· Losing control of your abdominals.
· Losing your imprinted pelvis position stability.
· Shortening the sides of your body while switching legs.

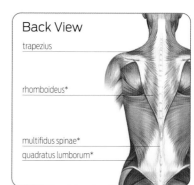

Back View
trapezius

rhomboideus*

multifidus spinae*

quadratus lumborum*

Annotation Key
Bold text indicates target muscles
Black text indicates other working muscles
* indicates deep muscles

Double-Leg Stretch

Double-Leg Stretch is the first of the classical Pilates stomach series. It works your powerhouse muscles, stretches your body, and develops coordination. Once you feel comfortable doing it along with Single-Leg Stretch, you will be able to easily flow between them. The closer your extended arms and legs are to the floor, the harder it is to stabilize your torso—so start by lowering only to the level that you can control comfortably.

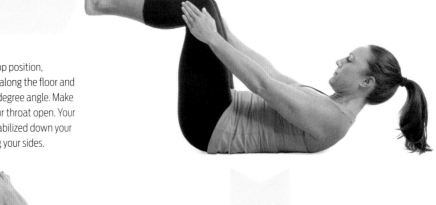

1 Lie on your back in tabletop position, with your spine extended along the floor and your bent legs forming a 90-degree angle. Make sure your neck is long and your throat open. Your shoulder blades should be stabilized down your back. Extend your arms along your sides.

2 Inhale as you begin to peel your upper body off the floor and forward toward your knees. Place your hands on the outsides of your calves.

Correct form
· Keep your abdominals flat throughout the exercise.
· Extend your legs only to an angle at which you can maintain torso stability.
· Keep your chin slightly tilted toward your chest.

Avoid
· Arching your back.
· Rolling your shoulders forward.
· Straining your neck.

3 Engage your lower abdominals, exhale, and lengthen your torso, extending your arms overhead to a position parallel to your ears. At the same time, extend your legs to a 45-degree angle above your mat.

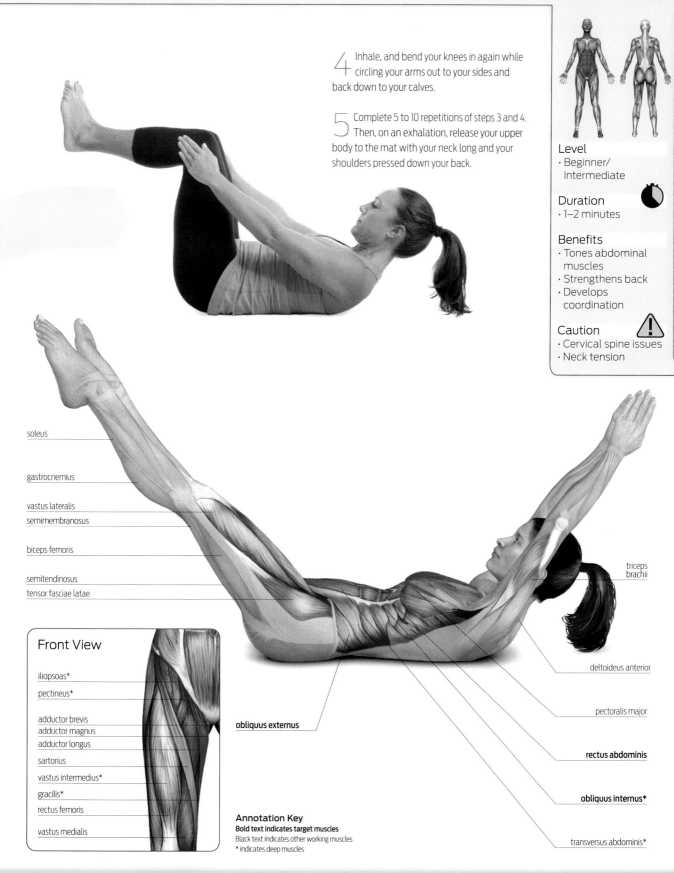

4 Inhale, and bend your knees in again while circling your arms out to your sides and back down to your calves.

5 Complete 5 to 10 repetitions of steps 3 and 4. Then, on an exhalation, release your upper body to the mat with your neck long and your shoulders pressed down your back.

Level
· Beginner/ Intermediate

Duration
· 1–2 minutes

Benefits
· Tones abdominal muscles
· Strengthens back
· Develops coordination

Caution
· Cervical spine issues
· Neck tension

soleus

gastrocnemius

vastus lateralis

semimembranosus

biceps femoris

semitendinosus

tensor fasciae latae

triceps brachii

deltoideus anterior

pectoralis major

rectus abdominis

obliquus internus*

transversus abdominis*

obliquus externus

Front View

iliopsoas*

pectineus*

adductor brevis
adductor magnus
adductor longus

sartorius

vastus intermedius*

gracilis*

rectus femoris

vastus medialis

Annotation Key
Bold text indicates target muscles
Black text indicates other working muscles
* indicates deep muscles

Spine Stretch Forward

Spine Stretch Forward increases the flexibility of your spine and stretches your hamstrings. It's one of those exercises where "less is more." If you don't feel an easy releasing sensation as you elongate your spine forward, take a moment to back up, adjust your alignment, and then try again.

1 Sit upright, with your arms down your sides, hands on the floor. Your legs should be extended in front of you, positioned hip-width apart with feet flexed. Inhale to prepare.

2 Exhale while pressing your navel to your spine and sequentially curling forward over your legs from your hip creases. Your arms should also move forward as your spine elongates over your legs.

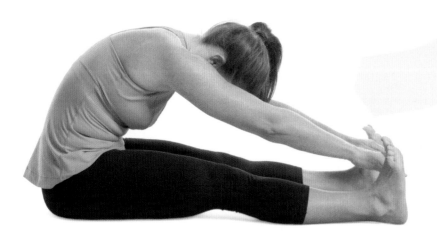

3 Maintain this position for 20 seconds, breathing deeply into your back and laterally into your rib cage.

4 On your last exhale, roll sequentially upward, from your tailbone and up through the tip of your head, until you are once more sitting upright.

Correct form
- Press your shoulders down and away from your ears throughout the exercise.
- Keep both sides of your neck long.
- Engage your lower-abdominal muscles.
- Anchor your legs along the mat.
- If your hips or hamstrings are tight, try sitting on a rolled-up towel.

Avoid
- Altering the position of your pelvis.
- Letting your knees roll inward.
- Holding your breath.

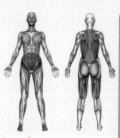

Modifications

Easier: Pressing your shoulder blades down your back, extend your arms up overhead, parallel to your ears. As you stretch your spine forward from your hip joints, lower your arms to shoulder height and hold. Imagine that someone is facing you, has taken your hands, and is gently pulling you toward them.

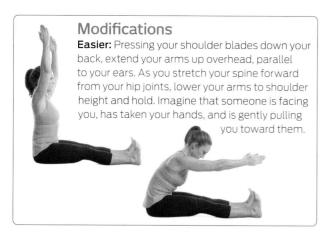

Annotation Key
Bold text indicates target muscles
Black text indicates other working muscles
* indicates deep muscles

Level
· Advanced

Duration
· 3–4 minutes

Benefits
· Improves spinal articulation
· Improves torso and leg flexibility
· Supports good posture

Caution
· Hamstring tightness
· Hip issues
· Knee issues
· Limited flexibility of the spine

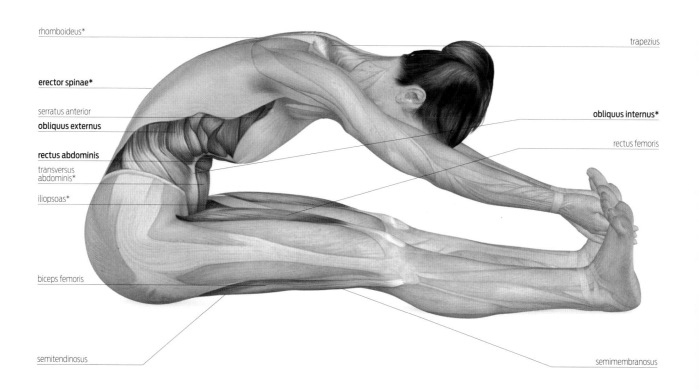

rhomboideus*

trapezius

erector spinae*

serratus anterior

obliquus externus

obliquus internus*

rectus femoris

rectus abdominis

transversus abdominis*

iliopsoas*

biceps femoris

semitendinosus

semimembranosus

Corkscrew

When practicing Corkscrew, it is important to keep your upper body perfectly stable while you describe precise circles in the air with your legs. Think of what you do when you use a corkscrew to open a bottle: you press down firmly (your torso) and rotate (your legs at your hip joints) simultaneously. The greatest challenge lies in keeping your shoulders pressed down your back and your pelvis anchored to the mat.

1 Lie on your back with your arms along your sides, palms downward for stability. Inhale to prepare.

2 While exhaling, imprint your spine, and lengthen your legs—one at a time—to the ceiling. Keep your legs parallel, firmly pressed together.

3 Stabilize your shoulder blades and your pelvis against the weight of your legs as you inhale and begin circling your legs to the right and down. Continue to circle your legs as you complete the circle on an exhalation.

4 Repeat, "drawing" a circle in the other direction. Complete 3 to 5 circles in each direction.

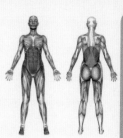

Front View

rectus abdominis

obliquus internus*

iliopsoas*

pectineus*

sartorius

rectus femoris

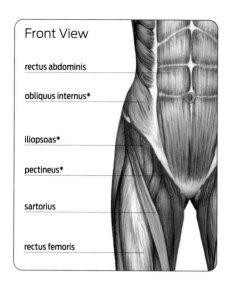

Level
· Intermediate/
  Advanced

Duration
· 1–2 minutes

Benefits
· Strengthens deep
  abdominals
· Increases upper
  body stability
· Improves hip
  mobility

Caution
· Hip issues or
  previous surgery
· Neck issues

transversus abdominis*

soleus

vastus lateralis

gastrocnemius

obliquus
externus

tensor
fasciae latae

semimembranosus

Correct form
· Keep your chest open and your shoulder
  blades pressed down your back.
· Anchor your whole spine into the mat.
· Keep your pelvis stable throughout the
  exercise.
· To prevent strain in your shoulders or hips,
  you can keep your knees slightly bent
  throughout the exercise if preferred.

Avoid
· Allowing your neck or back to arch.
· Rolling your shoulders forward.
· Releasing your abdominals.
· Losing energy in your legs.
· Making circles larger than you can control
  with your core muscles.
· Holding your breath.

Annotation Key
Bold text indicates target muscles
Black text indicates other working muscles
* indicates deep muscles

The Saw

The Saw is all about oppositions in space. You're twisting, flexing, and curving—all at once—while, of course, breathing calmly and fully. The goal of this exercise is to stretch your spine, sides, inner thighs, and hamstrings, while stabilizing your pelvis and shoulder blades. This is an exercise that feels great when you get the hang of it.

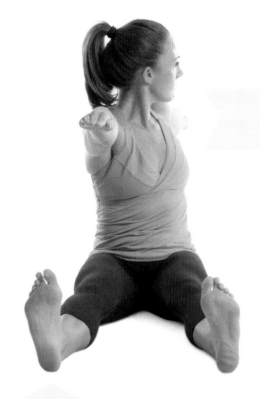

1 Sit upright, with your legs extended in front of you, a little wider than hip-distance apart. Flex your feet, pushing out through your heels to fully engage your legs. Extend your arms out to your sides so that they are parallel to the floor, palms down.

2 Pressing your navel to your spine, inhale while rotating around your vertical axis to the left, stretching your arms from under your shoulder blades and out through your fingertips.

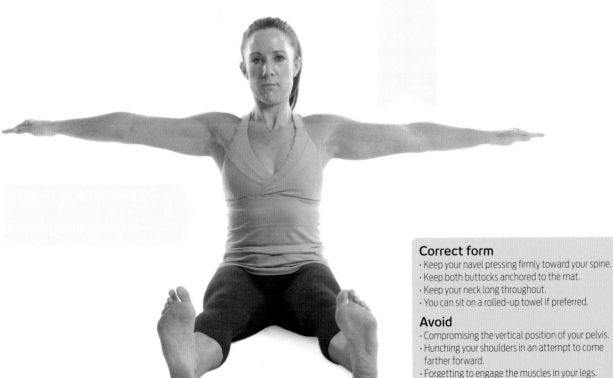

Correct form
· Keep your navel pressing firmly toward your spine.
· Keep both buttocks anchored to the mat.
· Keep your neck long throughout.
· You can sit on a rolled-up towel if preferred.

Avoid
· Compromising the vertical position of your pelvis.
· Hunching your shoulders in an attempt to come farther forward.
· Forgetting to engage the muscles in your legs.

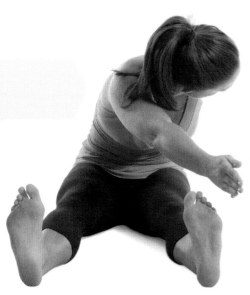

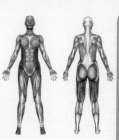

Level
· Intermediate/
Advanced

Duration
· 2–3minutes

Benefits
· Streamlines waistline
· Stretches hamstrings
· Enhances spinal
rotation and
flexibility

Caution
· Back issues
· Hip joint tightness
· Neck issues
· Shoulder issues

3 Exhale and rotate further to the left—and even further—in a twist out over your left leg, so that the pinky of your right hand "saws off" your little toe. At the same time, rotate your left arm—which is extending diagonally behind you—inward from your shoulder blade. Keeping both sides of your neck long, look toward that back arm.

4 As you inhale, roll up to your vertical twisted position again.

5 Exhale and face forward, returning to your starting position.

6 Repeat to the other side. Alternating, complete 3 to 5 repetitions to each side.

Annotation Key
Bold text indicates target muscles
Black text indicates other working muscles
* indicates deep muscles

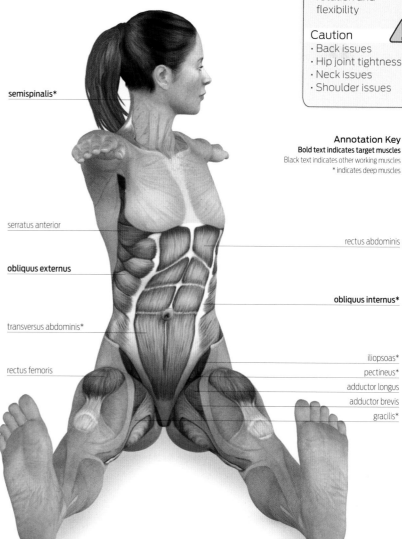

semispinalis*

serratus anterior

obliquus externus

transversus abdominis*

rectus femoris

rectus abdominis

obliquus internus*

iliopsoas*
pectineus*
adductor longus
adductor brevis
gracilis*

Back View

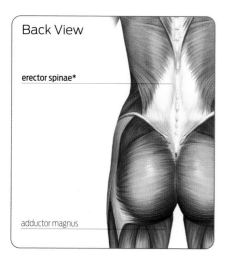

erector spinae*

adductor magnus

Neck Pull

Neck Pull works your abdominal strength, core stability, and spinal articulation while also stretching your hamstrings. The key to this exercise is to maintain a compact, stable, and anchored lower body.

Here's the challenge: your spine is going to roll, stretch, and hinge backward. Remain aware of what's going on with your back as you move through the positions.

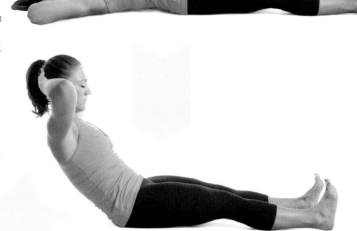

1 Lie on your back, with your pelvis and spine in neutral. Place one hand on top of the other beneath the base of your head. Extend your legs in front of you, hip-distance apart.
Flex your feet, engaging the muscles of your legs as you press your heels forward.

2 Inhale as you engage your abdominals, pressing navel to spine. Roll up from your mat one vertebra at a time, passing through the imprinted position to support this upward roll. Keep your legs firmly planted into your mat.

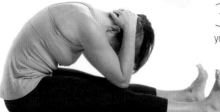

3 Exhale to lengthen your spine forward over your legs, keeping your elbows wide and your shoulders pressed down your back.

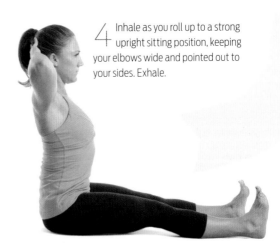

4 Inhale as you roll up to a strong upright sitting position, keeping your elbows wide and pointed out to your sides. Exhale.

Correct form
· Keep all movement smooth and elastic.
· "Button" both sides of your rib cage before beginning your upward roll.
· Engage your lower abdominal muscles when you curl up and curl down.
· Keep your neck long and throat open.
· Initiate all movement from your core, rather than from your extremities.

Avoid
· Tensing your neck, shoulders, or toes.
· Losing the position of your elbows.
· Losing connection with your legs.

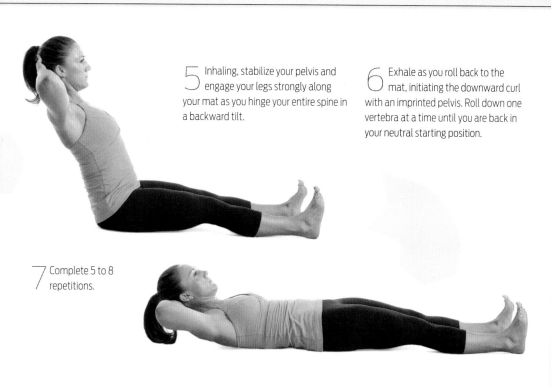

5 Inhaling, stabilize your pelvis and engage your legs strongly along your mat as you hinge your entire spine in a backward tilt.

6 Exhale as you roll back to the mat, initiating the downward curl with an imprinted pelvis. Roll down one vertebra at a time until you are back in your neutral starting position.

7 Complete 5 to 8 repetitions.

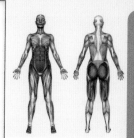

Level
· Intermediate/ Advanced

Duration
· 2–3 minutes

Benefits
· Develops abdominal strength
· Promotes spinal articulation, flexibility, and strength
· Improves posture

Caution
· Neck issues
· Spine issues

Annotation Key
Bold text indicates target muscles
Black text indicates other working muscles
* indicates deep muscles

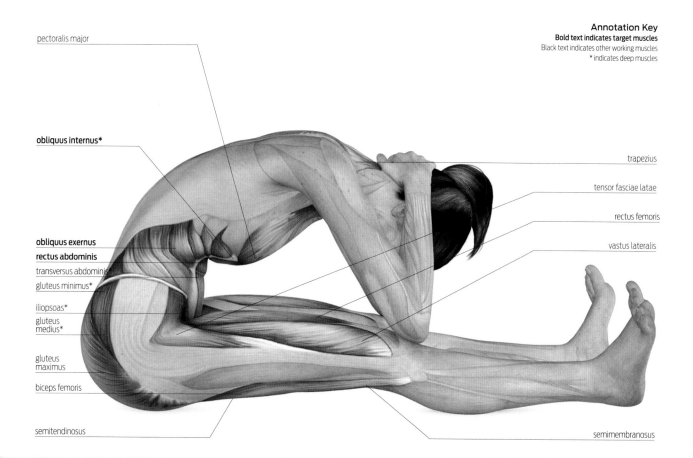

pectoralis major

obliquus internus*

obliquus exernus
rectus abdominis
transversus abdominis
gluteus minimus*
iliopsoas*
gluteus medius*
gluteus maximus
biceps femoris
semitendinosus

trapezius
tensor fasciae latae
rectus femoris
vastus lateralis
semimembranosus

The Scissors

In this exercise, your legs act as the blades of a pair of scissors. Use this image to perform precise, clear movements that cut through the air. Your core is the handle of the scissors that remains firmly in place, so that the blades are free to do their job.

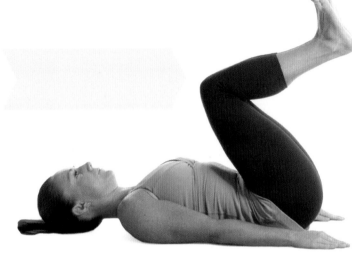

1 Lie on your back, with your pelvis in an imprinted position, your arms along your sides, and your knees folded in toward your chest.

2 Inhale as you curl your head and neck off your mat, extending your legs to the ceiling one at a time. Both buttocks should remain anchored to your mat throughout the exercise.

3 Exhale, and extend your arms toward your left leg so you can grasp it with both hands while the leg remains straight. At the same time, lower your right leg halfway to your mat.

4 Inhale and begin to switch legs by reaching both of them up to the ceiling so that they cross each other in mid-air.

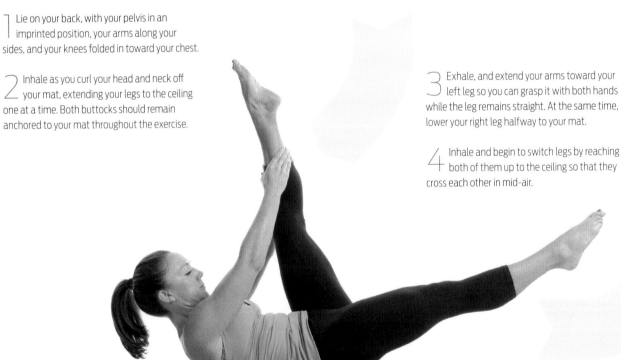

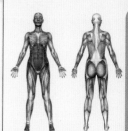

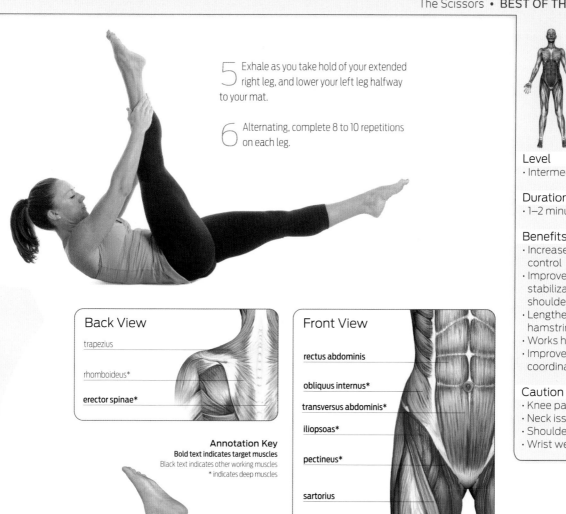

5 Exhale as you take hold of your extended right leg, and lower your left leg halfway to your mat.

6 Alternating, complete 8 to 10 repetitions on each leg.

Level
· Intermediate

Duration
· 1–2 minutes

Benefits
· Increases abdominal control
· Improves stabilization through shoulder area
· Lengthens hamstrings
· Works hip flexors
· Improves coordination

Caution
· Knee pain
· Neck issues
· Shoulder issues
· Wrist weakness

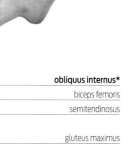

Back View
trapezius

rhomboideus*

erector spinae*

Front View
rectus abdominis

obliquus internus*

transversus abdominis*

iliopsoas*

pectineus*

sartorius

rectus femoris

Annotation Key
Bold text indicates target muscles
Black text indicates other working muscles
* indicates deep muscles

semimembranosus

serratus anterior

obliquus externus

obliquus internus*

biceps femoris

semitendinosus

gluteus maximus

Shoulder Bridge

Shoulder Bridge is one of those exercises that you'll find included in a variety of fitness and health programs, ranging from meditative yoga to elementary school calisthenics. Before you throw yourself into it, take an extra moment to read through this page in order to understand the Bridge from a Pilates point of view.

1 Lie on your back, with your pelvis and spine in neutral and your legs bent with feet on the floor. Your knees should be aligned with your hips and feet. Your feet should be fairly close to your buttocks, and firmly planted on the mat. Extend your arms along your sides, palms downward, and press your shoulders down your back to stabilize your shoulder blades. Inhale to prepare.

2 Exhale and curl your hips upward from the mat, creating a stable bridge position from your shoulders to your parallel knees. Holding this position, inhale.

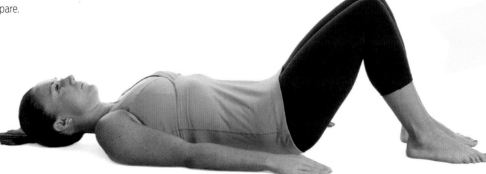

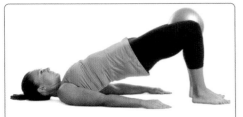

Modifications

Harder: Place a Pilates ball between your knees, squeezing it as you perform Shoulder Bridge. This modification increases lower-body resistance and enhances your awareness of the physical interconnections involved in the movement.

Correct form
· Maintain strongly engaged lower abdominal muscles.
· Keep your inner thighs active to maintain your parallel leg position.
· Keep your hips level.

Avoid
· Jamming your chin into your chest.
· Letting your rib cage "pop" forward and upward.
· Arching, and pushing into, your lower back while in the bridge.

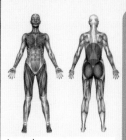

3 Exhale as you curl your spine back toward the mat, starting with your cervical vertebrae and rolling down your thoracic vertebrae and farther down to your lumbar vertebrae.

4 Repeat 3 times.

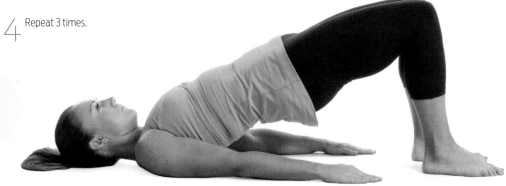

Level
· Beginner

Duration
· 2–3 minutes

Benefits
· Increases shoulder stability
· Strengthens powerhouse muscles
· Opens chest and pelvic area
· Works backs of legs

Caution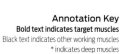
· Back injury
· Neck issues
· Shoulder issues

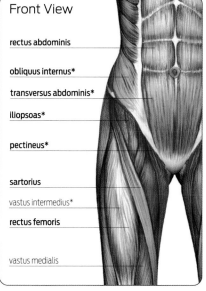

Front View

rectus abdominis

obliquus internus*

transversus abdominis*

iliopsoas*

pectineus*

sartorius

vastus intermedius*

rectus femoris

vastus medialis

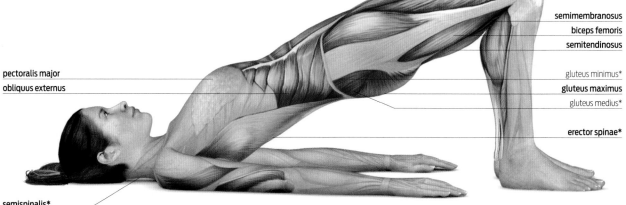

vastus lateralis

semimembranosus
biceps femoris
semitendinosus

gluteus minimus*
gluteus maximus
gluteus medius*

erector spinae*

pectoralis major
obliquus externus

semispinalis*

Side Leg Kick

Side Leg Kick is the first of a group of exercises done lying on your side. These exercises are quite tricky because you need to use your core stability and awareness of proper alignment in order to remain balanced.

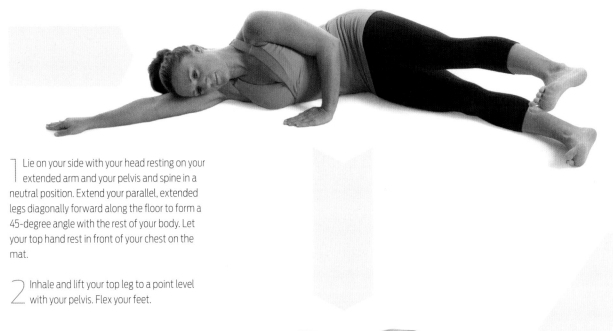

1 Lie on your side with your head resting on your extended arm and your pelvis and spine in a neutral position. Extend your parallel, extended legs diagonally forward along the floor to form a 45-degree angle with the rest of your body. Let your top hand rest in front of your chest on the mat.

2 Inhale and lift your top leg to a point level with your pelvis. Flex your feet.

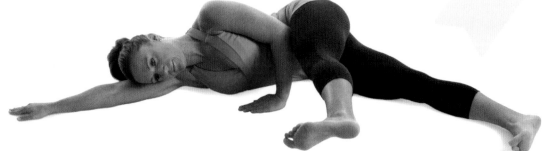

3 Exhale and, hinging from your hip joint, kick your top leg forward with the foot flexed.

Correct form
· Keep your pelvis and spine in place at all times.
· Brush your leg backward and forward to the same degree.
· Keep your shoulder blades pressed down your back.

Avoid
· Lowering your top leg as you swing it forward and backward.
· Rotating your hips.
· Bending your knees.

4 Inhale and, hinging from your hip joint, kick your top leg back with the foot extended.

5 Complete 8 to 10 repetitions. Switch sides and repeat with the other leg.

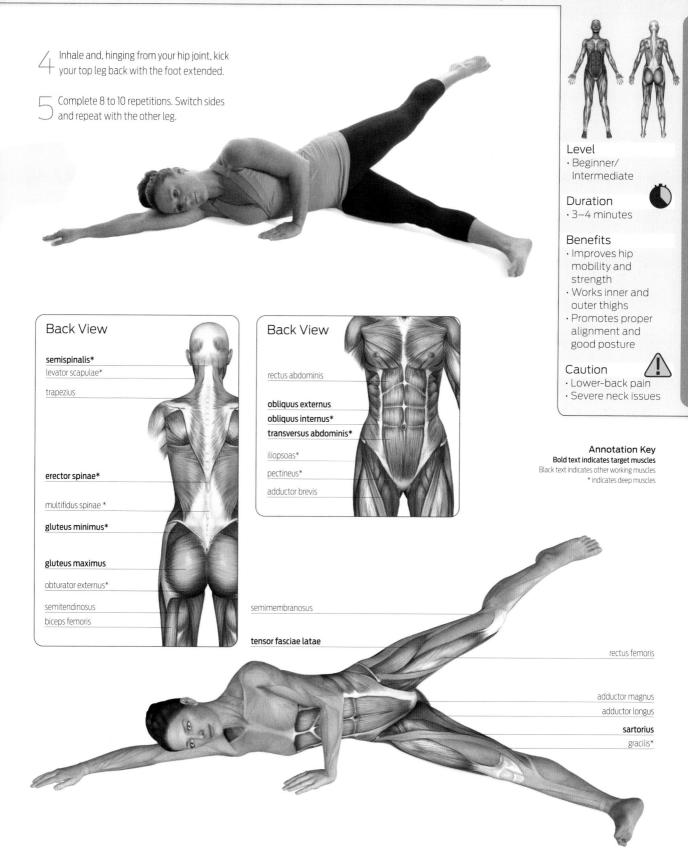

Level
· Beginner/ Intermediate

Duration
· 3–4 minutes

Benefits
· Improves hip mobility and strength
· Works inner and outer thighs
· Promotes proper alignment and good posture

Caution
· Lower-back pain
· Severe neck issues

Back View

semispinalis*
levator scapulae*
trapezius

erector spinae*

multifidus spinae *

gluteus minimus*

gluteus maximus

obturator externus*

semitendinosus
biceps femoris

Back View

rectus abdominis

obliquus externus
obliquus internus*
transversus abdominis*

iliopsoas*

pectineus*

adductor brevis

Annotation Key
Bold text indicates target muscles
Black text indicates other working muscles
* indicates deep muscles

semimembranosus

tensor fasciae latae

rectus femoris

adductor magnus
adductor longus

sartorius
gracilis*

Teaser Prep

Through regularly practicing Teaser Prep, you will find that your abdominal muscles become stronger, making the exercise's upward motion smoother and easier. It's a great way to prepare your core muscles, as well as the rest of your body, for the demands of the highly challenging Teaser (pages 60–61).

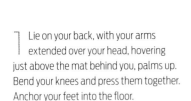

1 Lie on your back, with your arms extended over your head, hovering just above the mat behind you, palms up. Bend your knees and press them together. Anchor your feet into the floor.

2 Slowly and with control, extend one leg, straightening it from your hip and out through your foot.

3 Initiating the movement from your lower abdomen, raise your torso to form a 45-degree angle with the floor as you bring your arms up and over your head to reach forward.

4 With control, curl your spine down to the floor as you bring your arms up overhead and behind you again, keeping your knees pressed together.

5 Complete 2 more repetitions. Then, repeat on the other side.

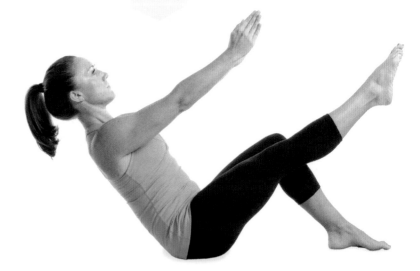

Correct form
· Keep your neck long and your throat open.
· Maintain a tight core and a level pelvis.
· When balancing, your arms should be parallel to your extended leg.

Avoid
· Arching your back or rolling your shoulders forward.
· Relying on momentum to propel you up or down.
· Allowing your stomach to bulge outward.

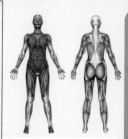

Front View

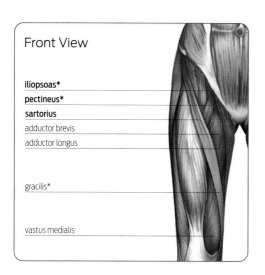

iliopsoas*
pectineus*
sartorius
adductor brevis
adductor longus

gracilis*

vastus medialis

Annotation Key
Bold text indicates target muscles
Black text indicates other working muscles
* indicates deep muscles

Level
· Intermediate

Duration
· 1–2 minutes

Benefits
· Strengthens and
  tones abdominals
· Mobilizes spine

Caution
· Herniated disc
· Lower-back issues
· Osteoporosis

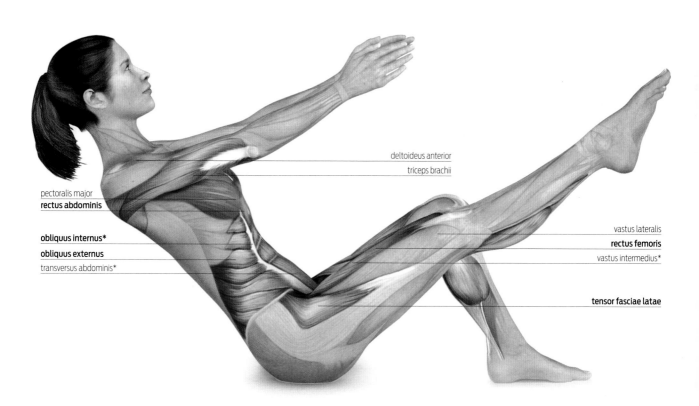

deltoideus anterior
triceps brachii

pectoralis major
rectus abdominis

obliquus internus*
obliquus externus
transversus abdominis*

vastus lateralis
rectus femoris
vastus intermedius*

tensor fasciae latae

Teaser

Teaser may be demanding, but it is also highly rewarding. Performing it successfully requires tuning in to your body's sense of balance, strength, coordination, and alignment. Don't worry if you find it difficult at first. With correct form, this exercise really works your powerhouse, effectively building your abdominal strength.

1 Lie on your back, with your arms extended over your head, hovering just above the mat behind you, palms up. Extend your legs on the mat in front of you so that your legs and torso form a straight line.

2 Initiating the movement from your lower abdomen, raise your torso to form a 45-degree angle with the floor as you bring your arms up and over your head to reach forward. Simultaneously, extend both legs forward to form a 45-degree angle with the mat. You should now be balancing on a point a couple of inches behind your sit bones.

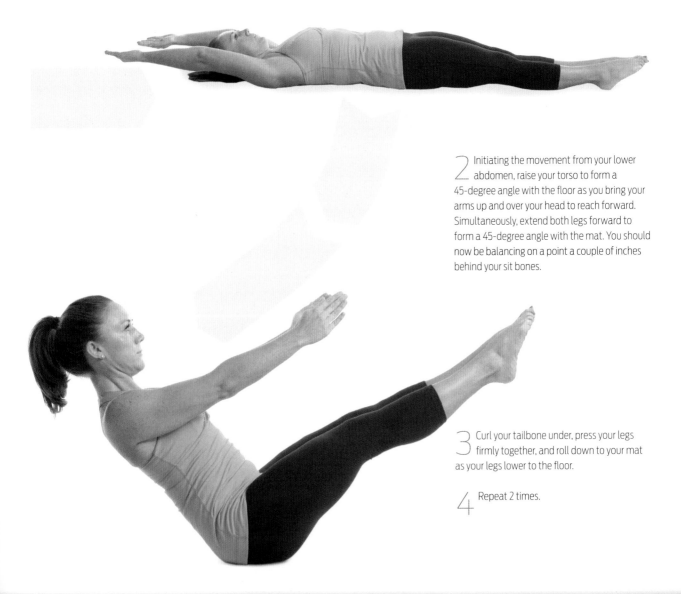

3 Curl your tailbone under, press your legs firmly together, and roll down to your mat as your legs lower to the floor.

4 Repeat 2 times.

Correct form
· Keep your legs together as if they were attached.
· Initiate movement from your lower abdominals.
· Keep your neck long and throat open.
· Maintain a tight core and a level pelvis.
· When balancing, your arms should be parallel to your legs.

Avoid
· Arching your back or rolling your shoulders forward.
· Using momentum to propel yourself up and down.
· Allowing your stomach to bulge outward.

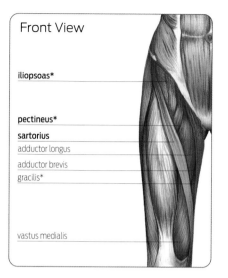

Front View

iliopsoas*

pectineus*

sartorius

adductor longus

adductor brevis

gracilis*

vastus medialis

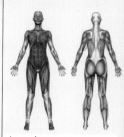

Level
· Advanced

Duration
· 2–3 minutes

Benefits
· Strengthens and tightens abdominals
· Mobilizes spine

Caution
· Herniated disk
· Lower-back issues
· Osteoporosis

Annotation Key
Bold text indicates target muscles
Black text indicates other working muscles
* indicates deep muscles

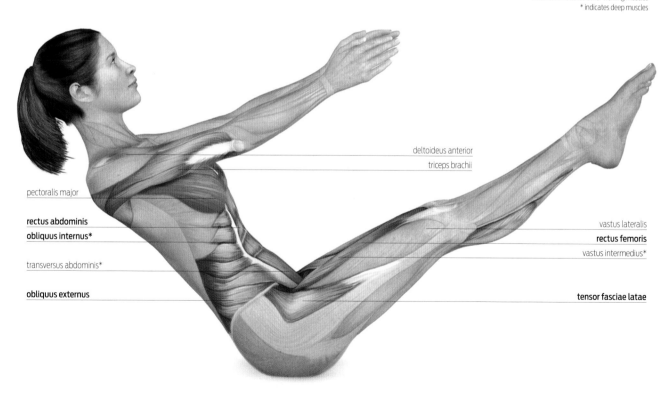

deltoideus anterior
triceps brachii

pectoralis major

rectus abdominis
obliquus internus*

transversus abdominis*

obliquus externus

vastus lateralis
rectus femoris
vastus intermedius*

tensor fasciae latae

Swimming

Swimming gets its names from the fluttering kicks in both legs and arms that resemble a body cutting through water. Like actual swimming, this exercise stretches and strengthens the muscles along your spine, and is good for your coordination, too.

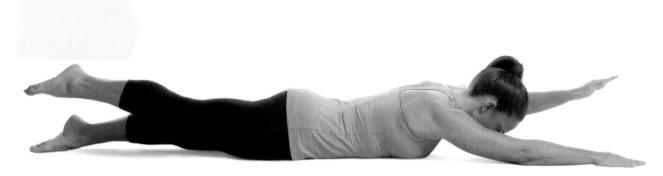

1 Lie on your stomach with your pelvis and spine in a neutral position. Extend your legs so that they're parallel and hip-distance apart. At the same time, extend your arms on the mat in front of you with your palms facing down. Keep your neck long and your face directed toward the mat. Press your shoulder blades down your back.

2 Inhale, and then press your navel to your spine while extending your arms in front of you and your legs behind you.

3 Exhale while continuing to extend your arms and legs until they lift slightly off your mat.

4 As you inhale for 5 counts, reach one arm and the opposite leg higher while lowering your other arm and leg—switching on every count. This is the "flutter kick."

5 Exhale for 5 counts as you continue to flutter your arms and legs in opposition and out into the space.

6 Repeat to complete 4 sets, which gives a total of 40 counts.

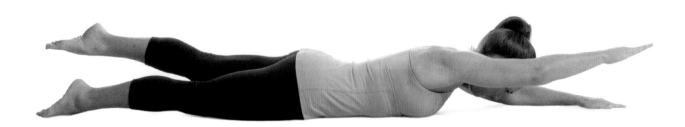

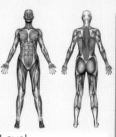

Back View

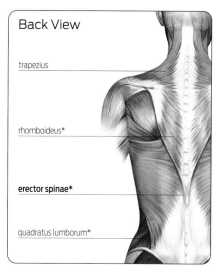

trapezius

rhomboideus*

erector spinae*

quadratus lumborum*

Back View

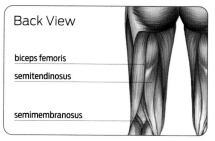

biceps femoris

semitendinosus

semimembranosus

Annotation Key
Bold text indicates target muscles
Black text indicates other working muscles
* indicates deep muscles

Level
· Beginner/
  Intermediate

Duration
· 2–3 minutes

Benefits
· Challenges core
  stability against
  dynamic movement
  of arms and legs
· Strengthens and
  stretches spine

Caution
· Cervical or lumbar
  spine curvature
· Lower-back issues
· Pregnancy

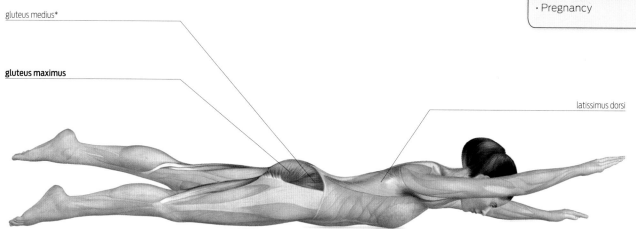

gluteus medius*

gluteus maximus

latissimus dorsi

Correct form
· Stabilize your shoulder blades by pressing your
  shoulders down your back.
· Keep your neck long and in alignment with the rest
  of your spine.
· Use your powerhouse to stay lifted.
· Keep the movements small and controlled.

Avoid
· Dipping your torso up and down as you "swim."
· Losing control of your legs as you move your arms.
· Letting your head and neck involuntarily react to
  the movements of your arms.

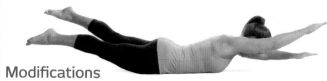

Modifications
Harder: You can increase the challenge of Swimming by elevating
your extended legs higher up from your mat. This vigorous
modification means that you'll have to provide extra support to
your lumbar spine by activating your abdominals down toward your
pelvis and back toward your spine. If you feel a pinching sensation
in your lower spine, or around your neck, lower your legs.

Leg Pull Front

Leg Pull Front is performed from a plank, or push-up, position, which is challenging to line up and maintain. Muscular length, strength, and movement flow are all worked thoroughly through this exercise.

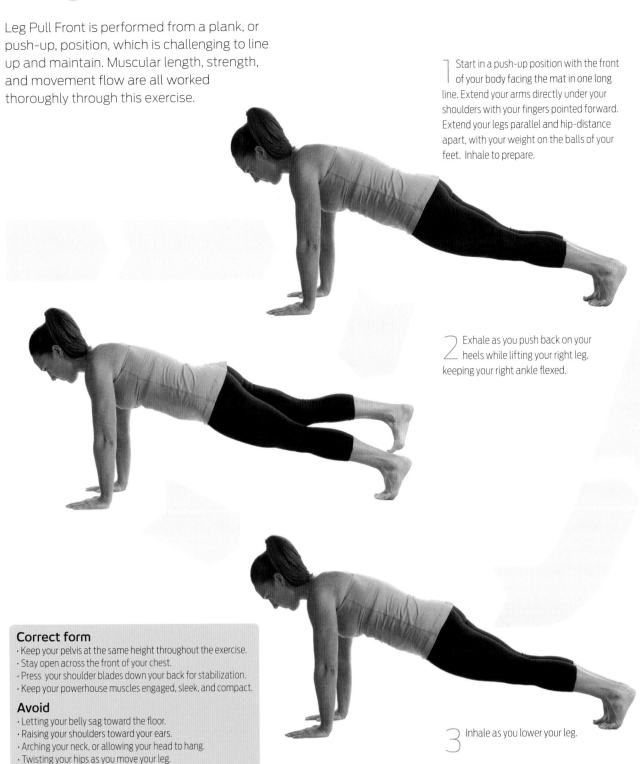

1 Start in a push-up position with the front of your body facing the mat in one long line. Extend your arms directly under your shoulders with your fingers pointed forward. Extend your legs parallel and hip-distance apart, with your weight on the balls of your feet. Inhale to prepare.

2 Exhale as you push back on your heels while lifting your right leg, keeping your right ankle flexed.

3 Inhale as you lower your leg.

Correct form
· Keep your pelvis at the same height throughout the exercise.
· Stay open across the front of your chest.
· Press your shoulder blades down your back for stabilization.
· Keep your powerhouse muscles engaged, sleek, and compact.

Avoid
· Letting your belly sag toward the floor.
· Raising your shoulders toward your ears.
· Arching your neck, or allowing your head to hang.
· Twisting your hips as you move your leg.

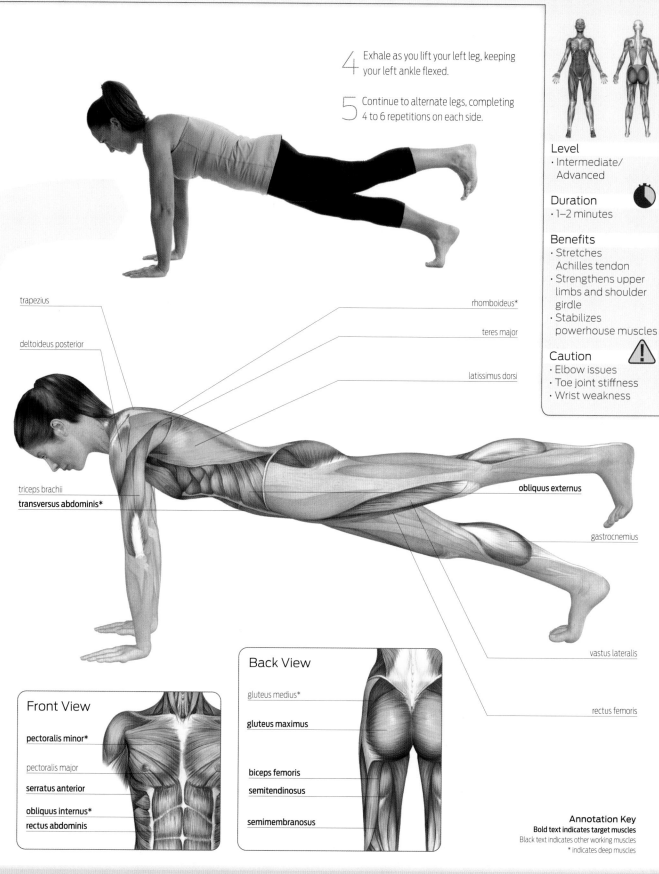

4 Exhale as you lift your left leg, keeping your left ankle flexed.

5 Continue to alternate legs, completing 4 to 6 repetitions on each side.

Level
· Intermediate/ Advanced

Duration
· 1–2 minutes

Benefits
· Stretches Achilles tendon
· Strengthens upper limbs and shoulder girdle
· Stabilizes powerhouse muscles

Caution
· Elbow issues
· Toe joint stiffness
· Wrist weakness

trapezius

rhomboideus*

deltoideus posterior

teres major

latissimus dorsi

triceps brachii

transversus abdominis*

obliquus externus

gastrocnemius

vastus lateralis

rectus femoris

Front View

pectoralis minor*

pectoralis major

serratus anterior

obliquus internus*

rectus abdominis

Back View

gluteus medius*

gluteus maximus

biceps femoris

semitendinosus

semimembranosus

Annotation Key
Bold text indicates target muscles
Black text indicates other working muscles
* indicates deep muscles

Side Leg Kick Kneeling

Side Leg Kick Kneeling is a more challenging variation on the Side Leg Kick exercise. It develops lateral strength in your torso and hip flexors, builds strength in your arms, and works your balance.

1 Kneel on your right knee on your mat. Make sure that your supporting right hand is on the floor directly under your shoulder. Extend your left arm to the ceiling. Extend your left leg, so that your foot is on the floor.

2 Inhale as you move your extended arm downward as your leg moves upward. Your leg and arm should meet precisely at the level of your hip.

3 Exhale as you reverse the movement to your start position.

4 You can either look forward or upward during the exercise. Choose the version that supports the elongation of your neck and an open position of your throat.

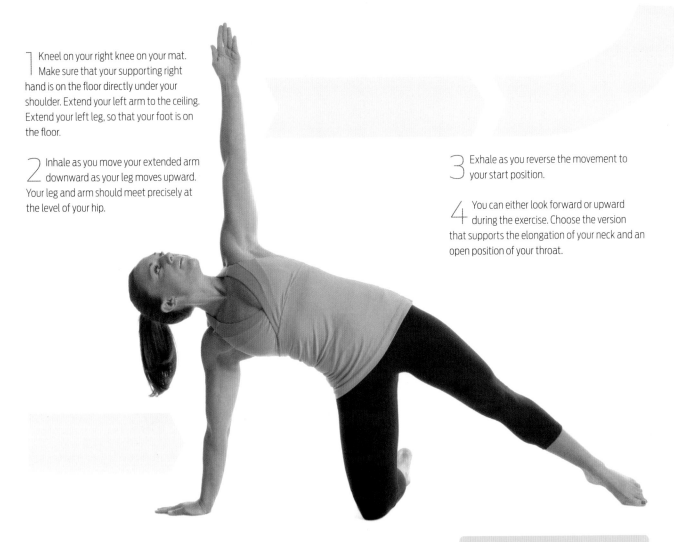

Correct form
· Keep both shoulders and your pelvis facing squarely forward.
· Lengthen away from your center.

Avoid
· Rolling your supporting arm forward.
· Locking the elbow of your supporting arm.
· "Popping" your rib cage forward.

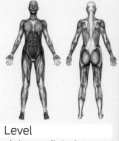

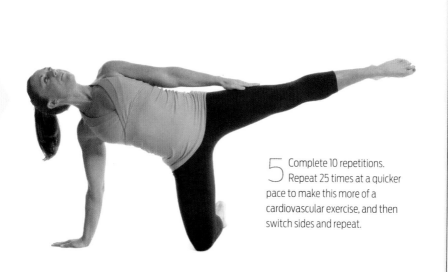

5 Complete 10 repetitions. Repeat 25 times at a quicker pace to make this more of a cardiovascular exercise, and then switch sides and repeat.

Level
· Intermediate/ Advanced

Duration
· 3–4 minutes

Benefits
· Develops torso stability
· Increases awareness of correct alignment
· Enhances ability to control legs from hip joints

Caution
· Knee issues
· Neck tension
· Shoulder injury

Back View

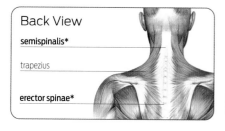

semispinalis*

trapezius

erector spinae*

Back View

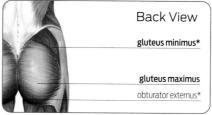

gluteus minimus*

gluteus maximus

obturator externus*

Annotation Key
Bold text indicates target muscles
Black text indicates other working muscles
* indicates deep muscles

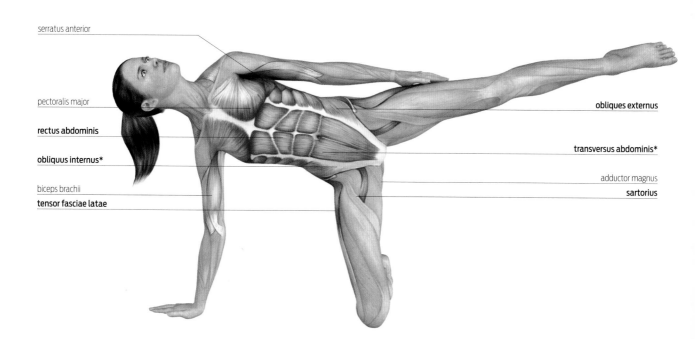

serratus anterior

pectoralis major

rectus abdominis

obliquus internus*

biceps brachii

tensor fasciae latae

obliques externus

transversus abdominis*

adductor magnus

sartorius

Side Bend

Side Bend is a great stretch that helps you to achieve a strong-as-steel powerhouse. Once you can do this exercise with relative ease, you know that you have truly come a long way!

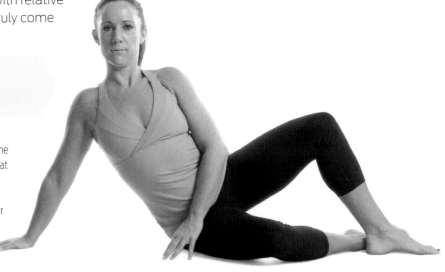

1 Sit on your right hip with your right arm supporting your torso, slighter away from the side of your body. Bend your right leg on the mat in front of you. Bend your left leg so that your knee points to the ceiling, your left foot flat on the mat slightly forward of your sit-bones. Your left arm should be on the mat in front of your right hip for balance.

2 Inhale as you begin to lift your pelvis, circling your left arm overhead and simultaneously straightening your legs. Lift higher in your hips so that your body creates a rainbow-like shape.

3 Exhale as you reverse the movement, so that you end up in your starting position sitting on the mat.

4 Repeat 3 to 5 times on one side. Then, switch sides and repeat.

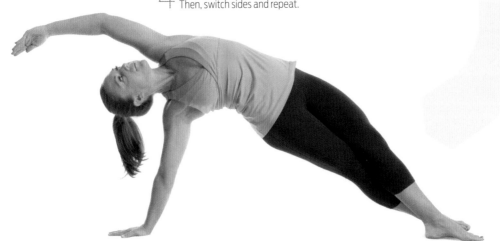

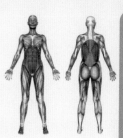

Correct form
- Adjust the distance of your feet to your pelvis while in the start position if you find that lifting to your side is difficult.
- Lift your hips high to reduce the weight on your supporting arm.
- Extend your arms and legs without locking either your elbows or knees.
- Keep your navel pressing to your spine.
- Use your abdominals and your breath to initiate movement.

Avoid
- Placing too much weight on your supporting arm.
- Sinking into your shoulders.
- "Popping" your rib cage forward.
- Rotating your hips.

Annotation Key
Bold text indicates target muscles
Black text indicates other working muscles
* indicates deep muscles

Back View

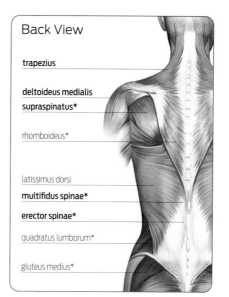

trapezius

deltoideus medialis
supraspinatus*

rhomboideus*

latissimus dorsi
multifidus spinae*
erector spinae*
quadratus lumborum*
gluteus medius*

Level
- Intermediate/ Advanced

Duration

- 3–4 minutes

Benefits
- Stabilizes spine in a neutral position
- Develops balance and proper alignment
- Strengthens torso, upper limbs, and oblique abdominal muscles
- Increases upper body flexibility

Caution ⚠
- Neck tension or stiffness
- Rotator cuff injury
- Wrist weakness

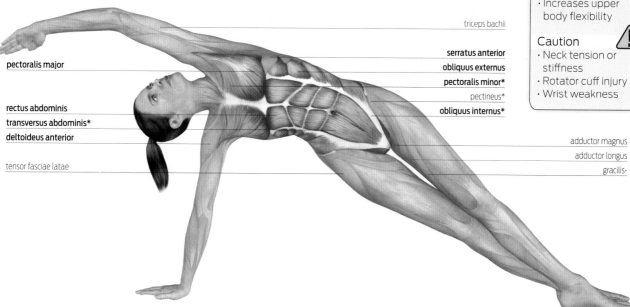

triceps bachii

serratus anterior
obliquus externus
pectoralis minor*
pectineus*
obliquus internus*

pectoralis major

rectus abdominis
transversus abdominis*
deltoideus anterior

tensor fasciae latae

adductor magnus
adductor longus
gracilis·

Modifications
Harder: Add an upper body twist to increase your thoracic spine rotation and stretch your rhomboid muscles. From your side bend extended position, rotate your upper torso to the right, so that your chest faces the mat—which will raise your hips even higher. Reach through with your left arm under your torso. Move through the basic side bend position from this rotation before returning to the start position again. Repeat on the other side.

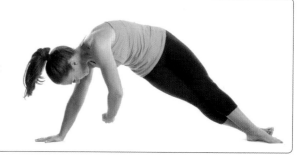

Push-Up

Push-Up, also known as a press-up, is a well-known calisthenics exercise performed everywhere: school gyms, Pilates and judo studios, and military boot camps, too. The reason for this is its effectiveness—it's a basic exercise that really works your chest, shoulders, back, and core.

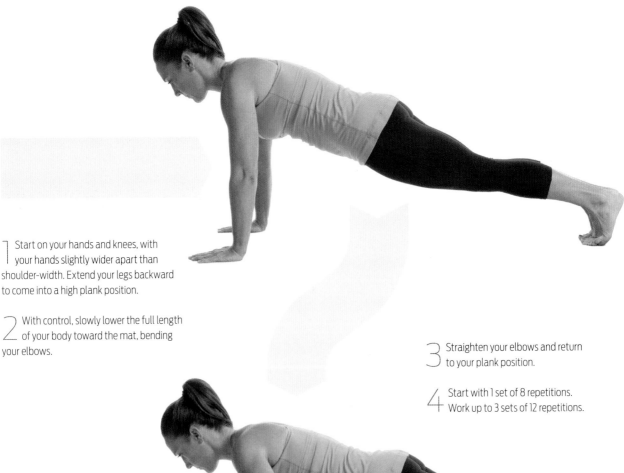

1 Start on your hands and knees, with your hands slightly wider apart than shoulder-width. Extend your legs backward to come into a high plank position.

2 With control, slowly lower the full length of your body toward the mat, bending your elbows.

3 Straighten your elbows and return to your plank position.

4 Start with 1 set of 8 repetitions. Work up to 3 sets of 12 repetitions.

Correct form
· Keep your shoulders pressed down your back.
· Imagine a straight line running from the top of your head to your heels.

Avoid
· Compromising the neutral alignment of your pelvis or spine.

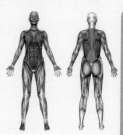

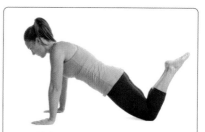

Front View

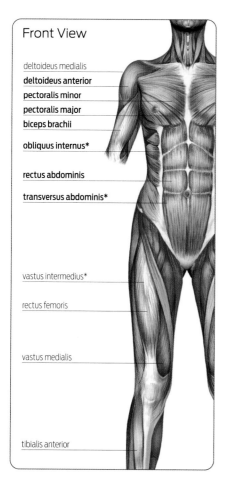

- deltoideus medialis
- **deltoideus anterior**
- **pectoralis minor**
- **pectoralis major**
- **biceps brachii**
- obliquus internus*
- **rectus abdominis**
- transversus abdominis*
- vastus intermedius*
- rectus femoris
- vastus medialis
- tibialis anterior

Modifications

Easier: Start on your hands and knees, with your hands slightly wider apart than shoulder-width. Lift your feet toward your buttocks until your calves and thighs form a 90-degree angle.

Level
- Advanced

Duration
- 2–3 minutes

Benefits
- Strengthens biceps, shoulders, chest, back, and core
- Tones abs

Caution ⚠
- Shoulder issues
- Wrist pain or other issues

Annotation Key
Bold text indicates target muscles
Black text indicates other working muscles
* indicates deep muscles

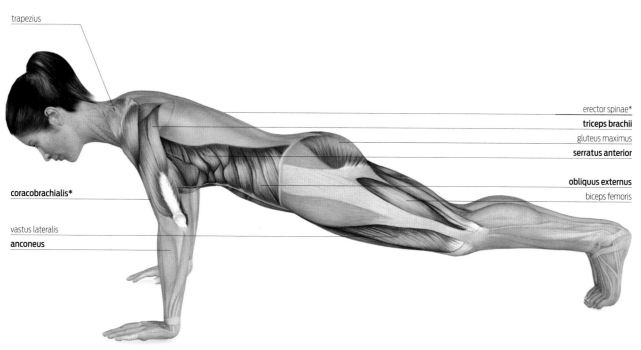

- trapezius
- coracobrachialis*
- vastus lateralis
- **anconeus**
- erector spinae*
- **triceps brachii**
- gluteus maximus
- **serratus anterior**
- **obliquus externus**
- biceps femoris

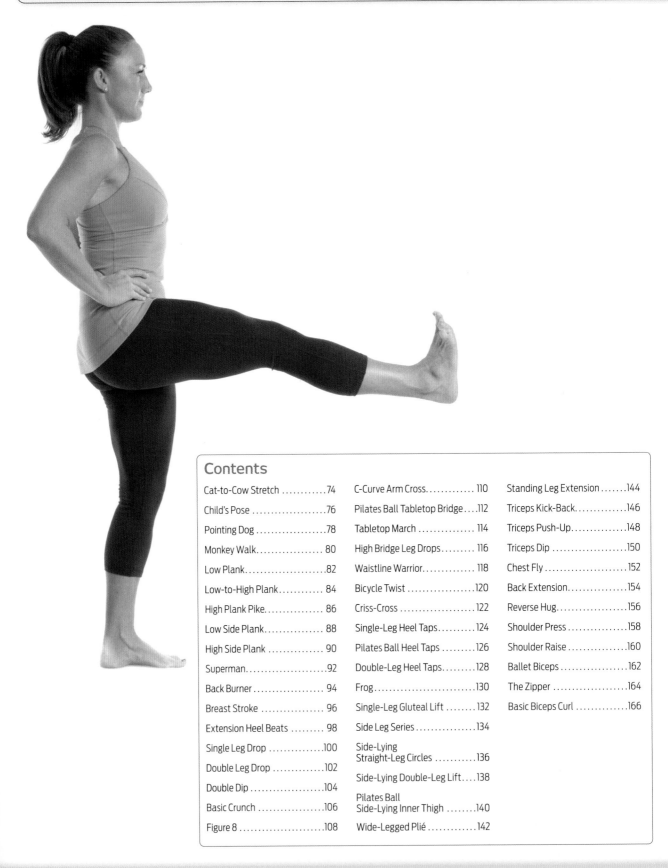

Contents

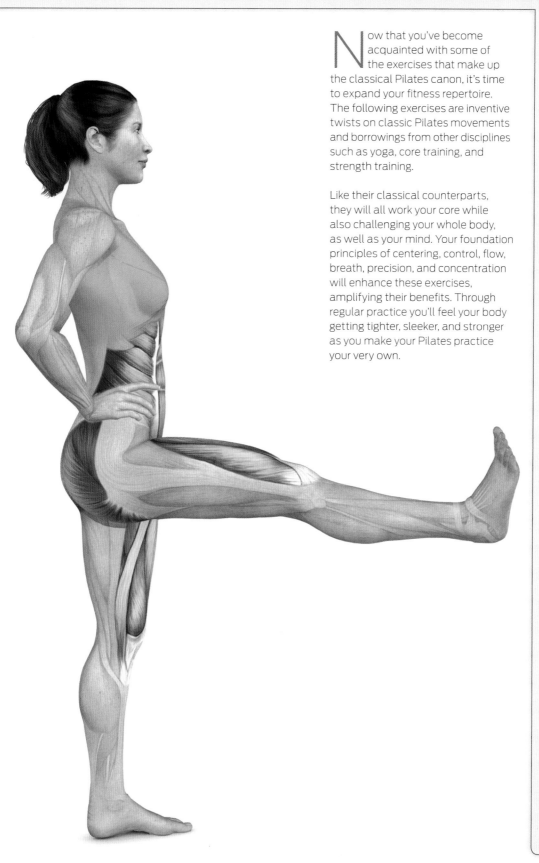

Now that you've become acquainted with some of the exercises that make up the classical Pilates canon, it's time to expand your fitness repertoire. The following exercises are inventive twists on classic Pilates movements and borrowings from other disciplines such as yoga, core training, and strength training.

Like their classical counterparts, they will all work your core while also challenging your whole body, as well as your mind. Your foundation principles of centering, control, flow, breath, precision, and concentration will enhance these exercises, amplifying their benefits. Through regular practice you'll feel your body getting tighter, sleeker, and stronger as you make your Pilates practice your very own.

Beyond the Classics

Cat-to-Cow Stretch

Also known as Cat and Dog, Cat-to-Cow Stretch is a great beginner's exercise, readying even the stiffest back for more strenuous activity. This is a feel-good exercise that warms up the entire spine.

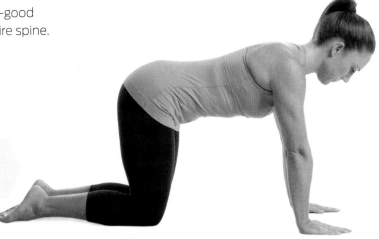

1 Kneel on all fours, with your knees directly below your hips. Position your hands on the floor just beyond shoulder-width apart, slightly in front of your body, palms downward and fingertips facing forward. Inhale as you press your navel back toward your spine.

2 Exhale as you sequentially curl your spine from your tailbone to your head. Your line of sight is now toward your navel.

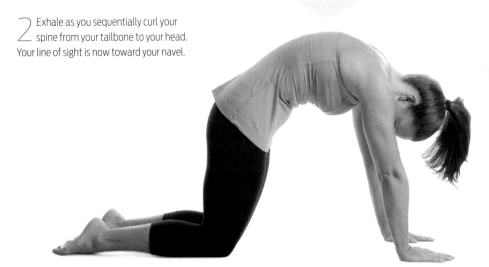

3 Inhale as you continue to expand the back of your rib cage, shoulders plugged down your back, and the sides of your neck extended long.

Correct Form
· Keep the sides of your neck long throughout the exercise.
· Engage your abdominals strongly and compactly.
· Maintain a parallel position of your arms and legs.

Avoid
· Lifting your shoulders toward your ears.
· "Popping" your rib cage.
· Closing your chest area.
· Arching primarily in your lower back.

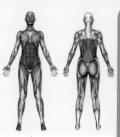

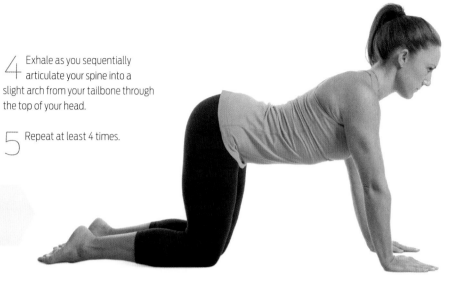

4 Exhale as you sequentially articulate your spine into a slight arch from your tailbone through the top of your head.

5 Repeat at least 4 times.

Level
· Beginner

Duration
· 1–2 minutes

Benefits
· Increases flexibility
· Improves balance and coordination
· Stretches spine, shoulders, hips, and abdominals

Caution
· Knee issues
· Wrist issues

Annotation Key
Bold text indicates target muscles
Black text indicates other working muscles
* indicates deep muscles

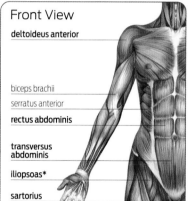

Front View

deltoideus anterior

biceps brachii
serratus anterior
rectus abdominis

transversus abdominis

iliopsoas*

sartorius

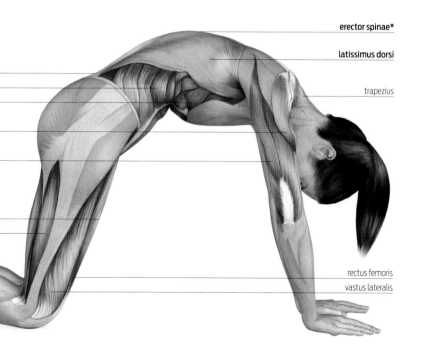

multifidus spinae*
obliquus externus
serratus anterior

deltoideus posterior

triceps brachii

vastus intermedius
biceps femoris

erector spinae*

latissimus dorsi

trapezius

rectus femoris
vastus lateralis

Child's Pose

Child's Pose is a resting position that you perform before, after, or while exercising. It's a back-releasing posture that elongates your spine and frees your shoulder blades from your rib cage.

1 Kneel on all fours, with your knees directly below your hips. Position your hands on the floor just beyond shoulder-width apart, slightly in front of your body, palms downward and fingertips facing forward. Inhale as you press your navel back toward your spine.

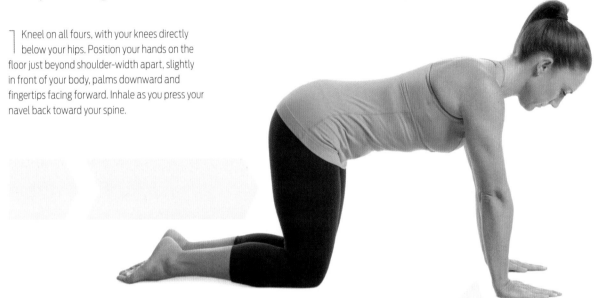

2 Sit back on your heels as you lower your chest onto your thighs with your arms extended in front of you on the mat. Your forehead rests on the mat and your knees and feet are together.

3 Breathe deeply into your pelvic area.

4 To come out of this position, exhale and use you abdominal muscles to uncurl your spine from your tailbone until you are sitting in a vertical position on your heels.

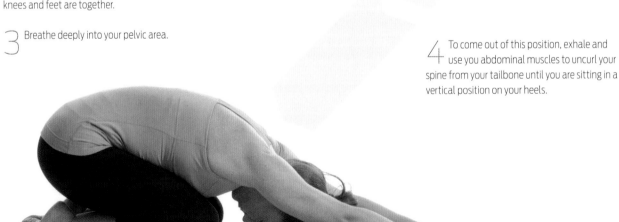

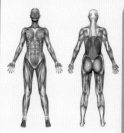

Correct form
· Keep your back rounded.
· Keep the sides of your neck long.

Avoid
· Compressing the back of your neck.
· Hunching your shoulders.

Modification

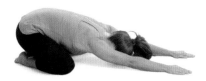

Same level of difficulty: With your feet still touching, widen your knees so your torso can release further down to the floor. Stay in this position for a while so that your body can deepen into a full stretch. The further apart your knees are, the greater the stretch in your inner thighs.

Level
· Beginner

Duration
· 5 seconds to 5 minutes

Benefits
· Stretches and relaxes the spine.
· Facilitates deep breathing into posterior ribs

Caution
· Knee issues

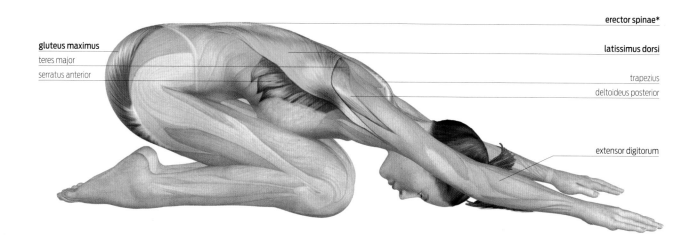

erector spinae*
gluteus maximus
teres major
serratus anterior
latissimus dorsi
trapezius
deltoideus posterior
extensor digitorum

Back View

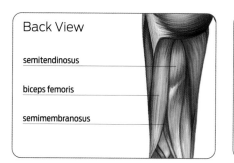

semitendinosus

biceps femoris

semimembranosus

Front View

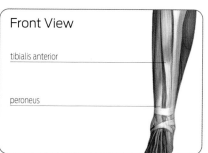

tibialis anterior

peroneus

Annotation Key
Bold text indicates strengthening muscles
Black text indicates stretching muscles
* indicates deep muscles

Pointing Dog

Pointing Dog, also know as Four-Point Challenge or Pointer, targets your abdominal muscles, buttocks, hamstrings, and lumbar spine. This exercise strengthens your lower back and the fronts of your thighs, and it is one of those "easier" exercises that challenges your balance, too.

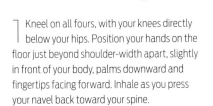

1 Kneel on all fours, with your knees directly below your hips. Position your hands on the floor just beyond shoulder-width apart, slightly in front of your body, palms downward and fingertips facing forward. Inhale as you press your navel back toward your spine.

2 With control, extend one leg directly behind you while extending the opposite arm in front of you. Hold this strong, level position for 2 to 5 seconds.

3 Return to the starting position, and repeat on the opposite side.

4 Complete a total of 10 repetitions (5 per side). Work up to 3 sets of 10.

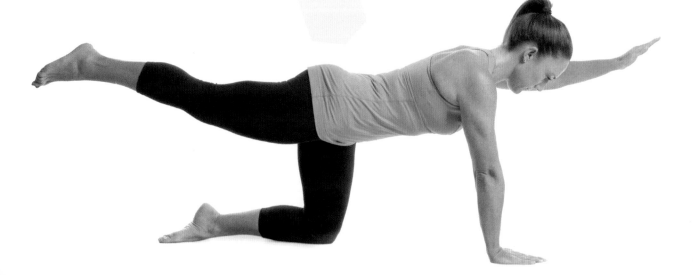

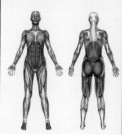

Back View

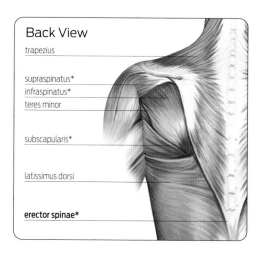

- trapezius
- supraspinatus*
- infraspinatus*
- teres minor
- subscapularis*
- latissimus dorsi
- **erector spinae***

Front View

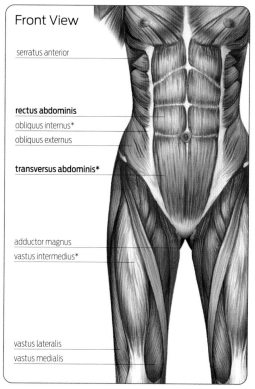

- serratus anterior
- **rectus abdominis**
- obliquus internus*
- obliquus externus
- **transversus abdominis***
- adductor magnus
- vastus intermedius*
- vastus lateralis
- vastus medialis

Level
· Intermediate

Duration
· 2–3 minutes

Benefits
· Strengthens abdominal, gluteal, and lower-back muscles
· Improves balance

Caution
· Back issues

Correct form
· Keep your abdominals fully engaged, navel pressing toward your spine.
· Press your shoulder blades firmly down your back.

Avoid
· Changing the level of your pelvis.
· Arching your neck.

Annotation Key
Bold text indicates target muscles
Black text indicates other working muscles
* indicates deep muscles

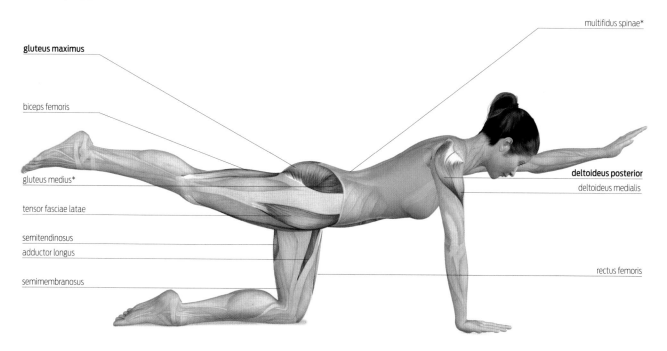

- multifidus spinae*
- **gluteus maximus**
- biceps femoris
- gluteus medius*
- tensor fasciae latae
- semitendinosus
- adductor longus
- semimembranosus
- **deltoideus posterior**
- deltoideus medialis
- rectus femoris

Monkey Walk

Monkey Walk is a good gauge of your fitness level—it's a full-body stretch that really tests the limits of your flexibility. If you are a beginner, you might find it difficult to keep your knees and back straight, but with practice, you can learn to smoothly move from one phase of the exercise to the next.

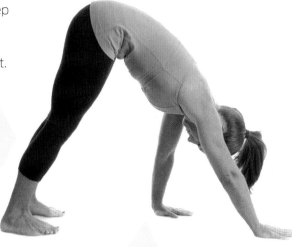

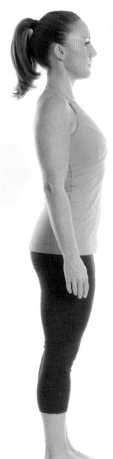

1 From a standing, parallel position, peel your spine downward toward the floor until your palms are flat on the floor in front of you..

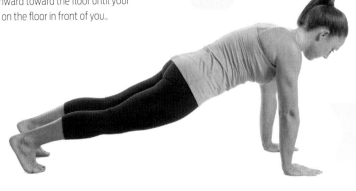

2 Slowly "walk" your hands out to a plank position with your wrists directly under your shoulders. Keep your body parallel to the floor, legs hip-width apart, navel pressing toward your spine and shoulders pressing down your back.

Correct form
· Widen your stance if you have trouble reaching the floor with your hands.
· Keep your abdominals sleek and compact.

Avoid
· Rushing through the exercise.
· Letting your stomach and spine sag while you're in the plank.

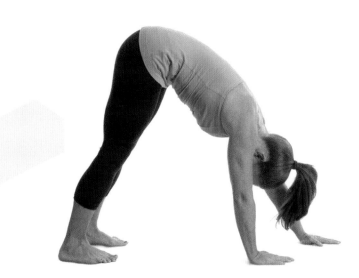

3 Pop your hips upward and push your weight back onto your heels. Your body should be in the shape of an upside-down V. Hold for a few seconds before slowly walking your hands back toward your legs.

4 Slowly release your spine upward, back to standing position. Pause, and repeat for 5 repetitions.

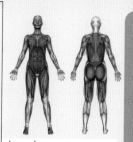

Level
· Intermediate

Duration
· 2–3 minutes

Benefits
· Stretches and warms up body
· Tones glutes and back

Caution
· Lower-back issues

Annotation Key
Bold text indicates target muscles
Black text indicates other working muscles
* indicates deep muscles

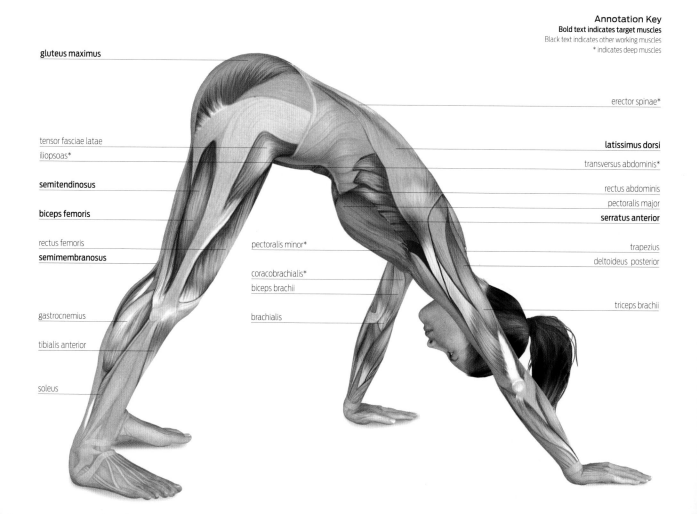

gluteus maximus

erector spinae*

tensor fasciae latae

latissimus dorsi

iliopsoas*

transversus abdominis*

semitendinosus

rectus abdominis

pectoralis major

biceps femoris

serratus anterior

rectus femoris

pectoralis minor*

trapezius

semimembranosus

deltoideus posterior

coracobrachialis*

biceps brachii

triceps brachii

gastrocnemius

brachialis

tibialis anterior

soleus

Low Plank

There are many versions of the plank, and they all work to tighten up your core and help you sense how interconnected and powerful your body actually is. Low Plank adds an extra challenge to your training because you have to maintain your core stability while you remain positioned just above your mat.

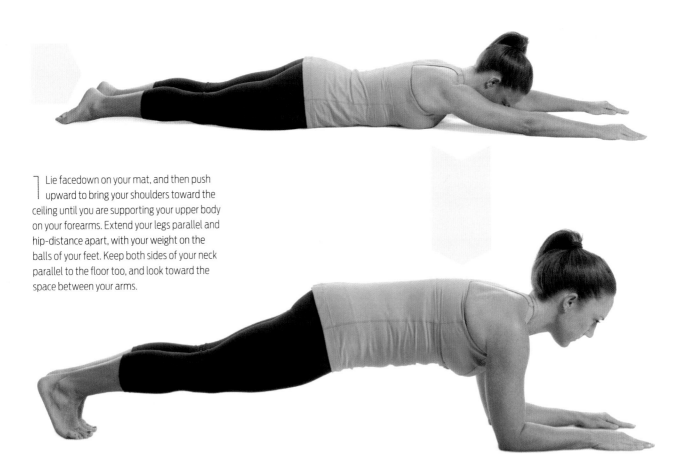

1 Lie facedown on your mat, and then push upward to bring your shoulders toward the ceiling until you are supporting your upper body on your forearms. Extend your legs parallel and hip-distance apart, with your weight on the balls of your feet. Keep both sides of your neck parallel to the floor too, and look toward the space between your arms.

2 Inhale for 5 counts, and exhale for 5 counts as you keep your shoulders gliding down your back and your navel pressing back toward your spine.

3 Complete 3 to 5 sets before releasing out of the position.

Correct form
· Lengthen through your neck.
· Stabilize your shoulders.
· Draw your rib cage down toward your pelvis.
· Lift up along your hamstrings.

Avoid
· Letting your stomach sag.
· Tensing your shoulders.
· Bearing too much weight on your elbows.

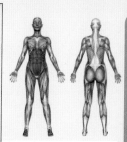

Front View

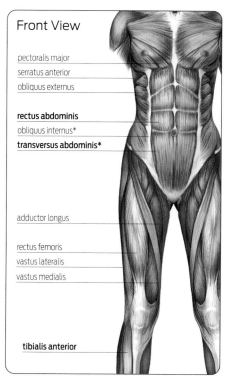

pectoralis major
serratus anterior
obliquus externus

rectus abdominis
obliquus internus*
transversus abdominis*

adductor longus

rectus femoris
vastus lateralis
vastus medialis

tibialis anterior

Back View

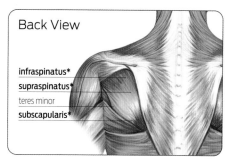

infraspinatus*
supraspinatus*
teres minor
subscapularis*

Annotation Key
Bold text indicates target muscles
Black text indicates other working muscles
* indicates deep muscles

Level
· Intermediate/
  Advanced

Duration
· 2–3 minutes

Benefits
· Strengthens and
  stabilizes core
· Strengthens
  abdominals

Caution
· Elbow injury
· Shoulder issues

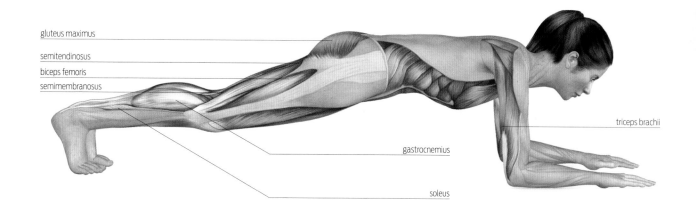

gluteus maximus
semitendinosus
biceps femoris
semimembranosus

gastrocnemius

soleus

triceps brachii

Modification

Harder: Keep your hips level and parallel to the floor.
Flex your right knee toward the mat as you
inhale and extend it again as you exhale.
Alternate sides, performing 2 to 4
sets on each leg.

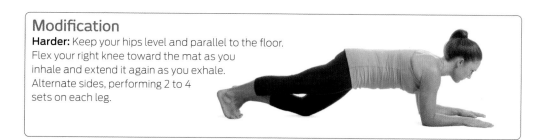

Low-to-High Plank

If you want to tone your abdominals and arms, then Low-to-High Plank will do the job. Focus on keeping your abdominals fully engaged as you move from low to high and back again.

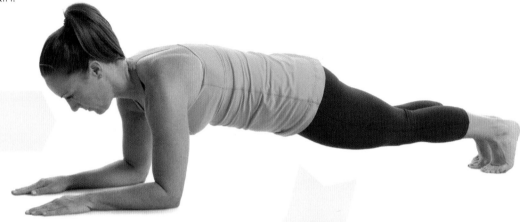

1 Start in Low Plank, with your weight evenly distributed on your elbows and the balls of your feet. Take a moment to stabilize your hips in this position and really engage your abdominals.

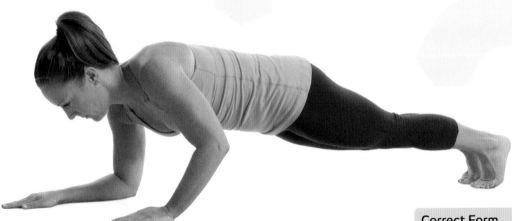

2 Reposition one arm and then the other so that your hands are on the mat in front of your shoulders, lifting your body into High Plank.

Correct Form
· Keep your navel pressed toward your spine for strength throughout the exercise.

Avoid
· Letting your stomach or rib cage sag.
· Lifting your shoulders up and/or forward.
· Shifting your weight when you change levels.

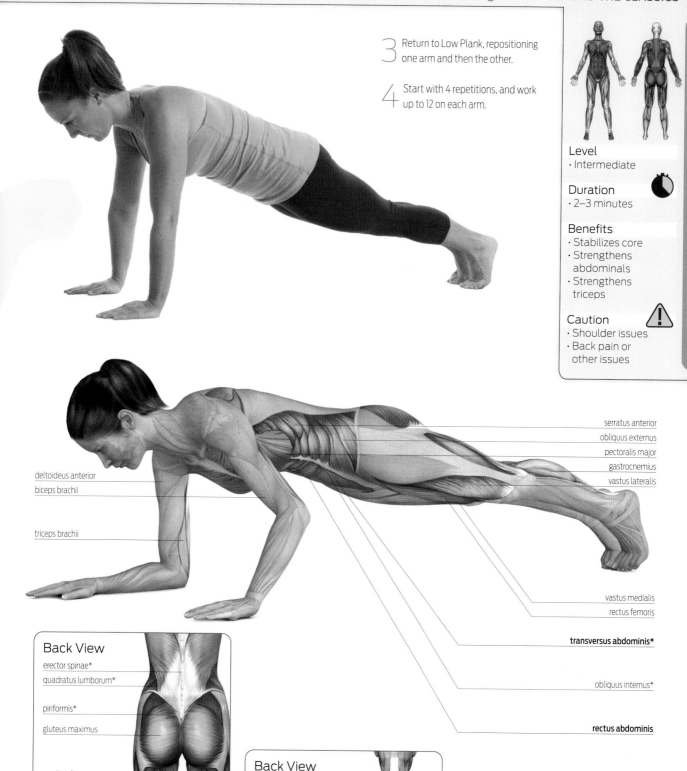

3 Return to Low Plank, repositioning one arm and then the other.

4 Start with 4 repetitions, and work up to 12 on each arm.

Level
· Intermediate

Duration
· 2–3 minutes

Benefits
· Stabilizes core
· Strengthens abdominals
· Strengthens triceps

Caution
· Shoulder issues
· Back pain or other issues

serratus anterior
obliquus externus
pectoralis major
gastrocnemius
vastus lateralis

deltoideus anterior
biceps brachii

triceps brachii

vastus medialis
rectus femoris

transversus abdominis*

obliquus internus

rectus abdominis

Back View

erector spinae*
quadratus lumborum*

piriformis*

gluteus maximus

semitendinosus

biceps femoris

semimembranosus

Back View

trapezius

deltoideus posterior

teres minor
teres major

Annotation Key
Bold text indicates target muscles
Black text indicates other working muscles
* indicates deep muscles

High Plank Pike

High Plank Pike combines the strength of the high plank position with the yoga "downward-facing dog" stretch. It increases strength in your upper limbs, chest, and upper back and increases flexibility in your spine, hip joints, and hamstrings.

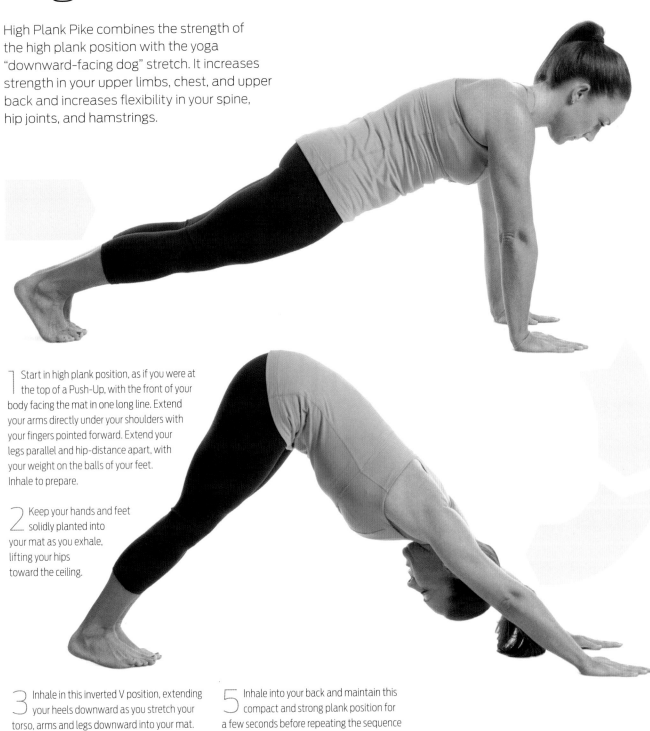

1 Start in high plank position, as if you were at the top of a Push-Up, with the front of your body facing the mat in one long line. Extend your arms directly under your shoulders with your fingers pointed forward. Extend your legs parallel and hip-distance apart, with your weight on the balls of your feet. Inhale to prepare.

2 Keep your hands and feet solidly planted into your mat as you exhale, lifting your hips toward the ceiling.

3 Inhale in this inverted V position, extending your heels downward as you stretch your torso, arms and legs downward into your mat.

4 Exhale as you return to the position.

5 Inhale into your back and maintain this compact and strong plank position for a few seconds before repeating the sequence 3 to 6 times.

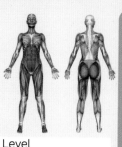

Correct Form
- Keep your shoulders plugged down your back.
- Maintain the length of your neck—and an open throat—throughout the exercise.
- Keep your body taut and your elbows close to your sides while in the plank position.
- Stretch your spine from your coccyx and out through the tips of your ears when you're in the inverted V shape.

Avoid
- Pressing into your lower back.
- Hunching your shoulders.
- Rolling your shoulders forward.
- Letting go of your abdominals.

Annotation Key
Bold text indicates target muscles
Black text indicates other working muscles
* indicates deep muscles

Level
- Intermediate

Duration
- 2–3 minutes

Benefits
- Works scapulae stabilizers
- Strengthens and stretches entire spine

Caution
- Shoulder issues
- Toe joint stiffness
- Wrist weakness

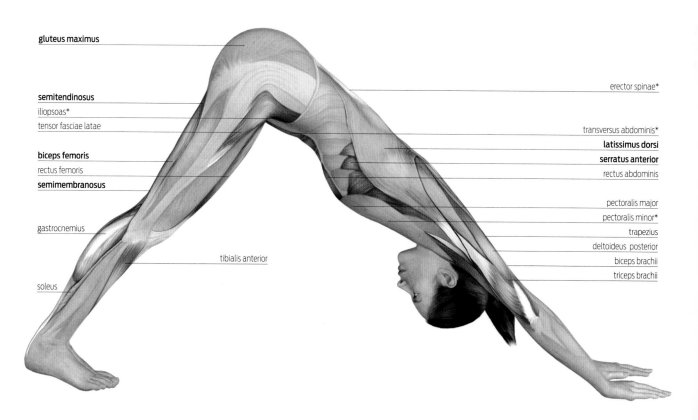

gluteus maximus

semitendinosus
iliopsoas*
tensor fasciae latae

biceps femoris
rectus femoris
semimembranosus

gastrocnemius

tibialis anterior

soleus

erector spinae*

transversus abdominis*
latissimus dorsi
serratus anterior
rectus abdominis

pectoralis major
pectoralis minor*
trapezius
deltoideus posterior
biceps brachii
triceps brachii

Low Side Plank

Low Side Plank develops your balance, and strengthens your torso, abdominals (especially the obliques), and upper limbs. Don't forget your legs, as they're the solid foundation that will make it possible to shift direction without losing control.

Correct Form
· Keep the sides of your neck long.
· Remain lifted out of your shoulder throughout the exercise.
· Raise your hips slightly to relieve pressure on your supporting arm.
· Pull up along the front of your hips and thighs.
· Keep your ankles strongly flexed.
· If you find it uncomfortable to turn your neck to face your extended top arm, gaze forward instead.

Avoid
· Lifting your shoulders.
· Letting your body weight sink into your supporting arms.

1 Assume a low plank position, with your body forming a straight line, your hands directly beneath your shoulders, and your feet planted hip-width apart. Place your weight on the balls of your feet, and inhale.

2 Exhale as you rotate your body to the left, extending your left arm toward the ceiling as your left leg comes to rest on top of your right. Turn your head upward to look toward your extended arm.

3 Lift your hips slightly higher as you press your navel to your spine. This will take some of the weight off your supporting arm. Inhale as you stabilize this position.

4 Rotate your body as you exhale, returning to your low plank again.

5 Complete 2 to 3 repetitions on one side, and then switch sides and repeat.

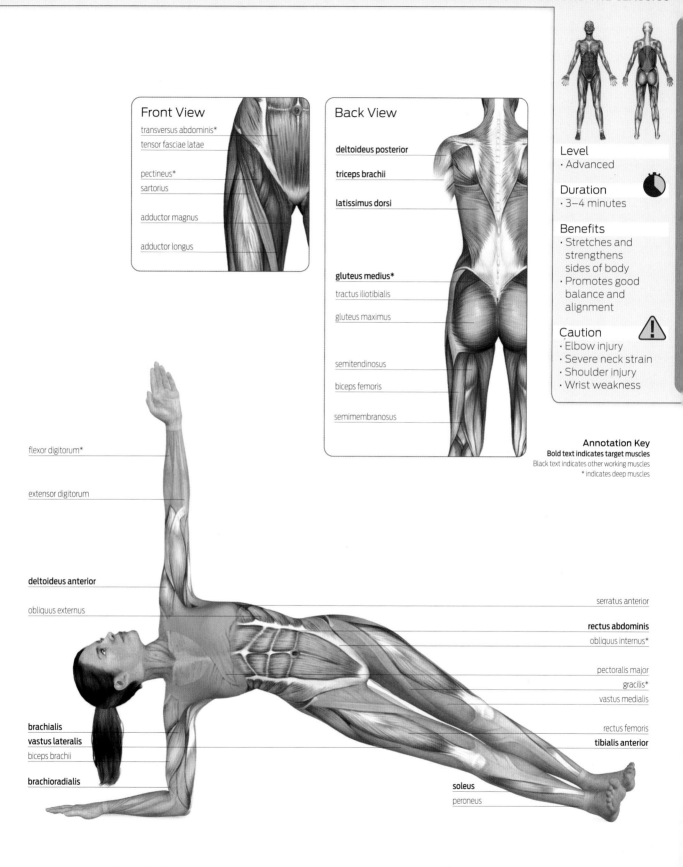

Front View

transversus abdominis*

tensor fasciae latae

pectineus*

sartorius

adductor magnus

adductor longus

Back View

deltoideus posterior

triceps brachii

latissimus dorsi

gluteus medius*

tractus iliotibialis

gluteus maximus

semitendinosus

biceps femoris

semimembranosus

Level
· Advanced

Duration
· 3–4 minutes

Benefits
· Stretches and
  strengthens
  sides of body
· Promotes good
  balance and
  alignment

Caution
· Elbow injury
· Severe neck strain
· Shoulder injury
· Wrist weakness

Annotation Key
Bold text indicates target muscles
Black text indicates other working muscles
* indicates deep muscles

flexor digitorum*

extensor digitorum

deltoideus anterior

obliquus externus

brachialis

vastus lateralis

biceps brachii

brachioradialis

serratus anterior

rectus abdominis

obliquus internus*

pectoralis major

gracilis*

vastus medialis

rectus femoris

tibialis anterior

soleus

peroneus

High Side Plank

High Side Plank is another variation on the plank exercise. In general, the plank exercises are great for increasing your endurance while challenging your powerhouse; if possible, try to include at least one variation every time you practice. This is a demanding exercise, so make sure that you are physically warm enough, as well as focused enough, to perform it properly.

Correct Form
· Lengthen through your neck.
· Lift up along the front of your pelvis and thighs.
· If you find it uncomfortable to turn your neck to face your extended top arm, gaze forward.
· Elongate your entire body.

Avoid
· Allowing your shoulders to move upward toward your ears.
· Letting your shoulders collapse into your shoulder joints.
· Twisting your neck.

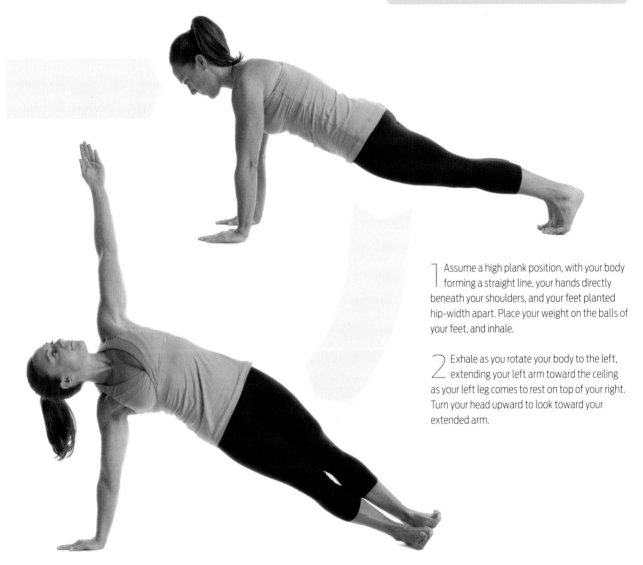

1 Assume a high plank position, with your body forming a straight line, your hands directly beneath your shoulders, and your feet planted hip-width apart. Place your weight on the balls of your feet, and inhale.

2 Exhale as you rotate your body to the left, extending your left arm toward the ceiling as your left leg comes to rest on top of your right. Turn your head upward to look toward your extended arm.

3 Lift your hips higher as you press your navel to your spine. Inhale into your pelvic area.

4 Rotate your body as you exhale, returning to your high plank position again.

5 Complete 2 to 3 repetitions on one side, and then switch sides and repeat.

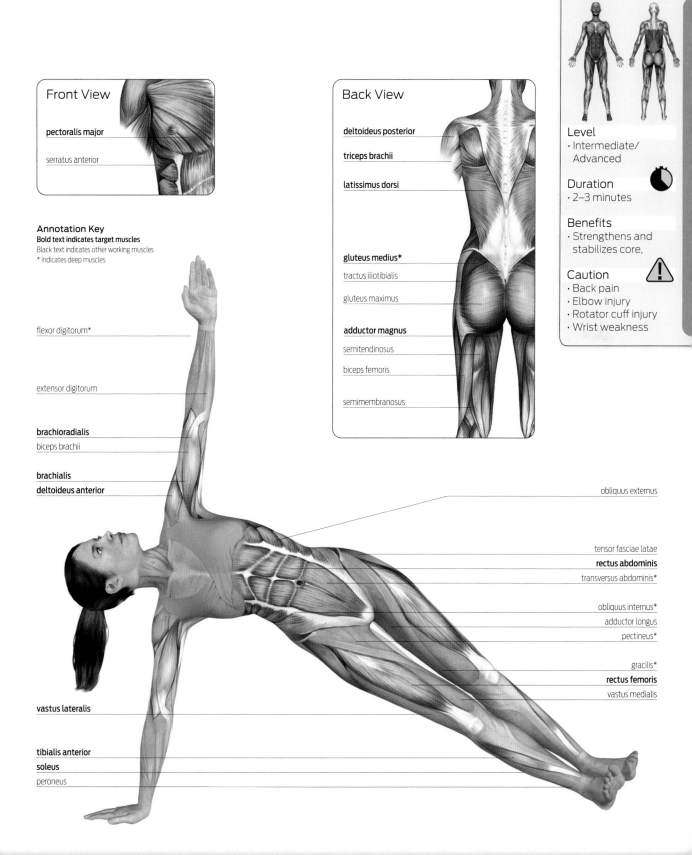

Front View

pectoralis major

serratus anterior

Back View

deltoideus posterior

triceps brachii

latissimus dorsi

gluteus medius*

tractus iliotibialis

gluteus maximus

adductor magnus

semitendinosus

biceps femoris

semimembranosus

Annotation Key
Bold text indicates target muscles
Black text indicates other working muscles
* indicates deep muscles

Level
· Intermediate/ Advanced

Duration
· 2–3 minutes

Benefits
· Strengthens and stabilizes core,

Caution
· Back pain
· Elbow injury
· Rotator cuff injury
· Wrist weakness

flexor digitorum*

extensor digitorum

brachioradialis
biceps brachii

brachialis
deltoideus anterior

obliquus externus

tensor fasciae latae
rectus abdominis
transversus abdominis*

obliquus internus*
adductor longus
pectineus*

gracilis*
rectus femoris
vastus medialis

vastus lateralis

tibialis anterior
soleus
peroneus

Superman

Like Swimming (pages 62–63) and Back Burner (pages 94–95), Superman really helps to elongate your spine and strengthen your spinal extensors. Even though you perform this exercise lying on your stomach, be sure to keep your rib cage zipped back toward your spine and your lower abdominals strongly engaged.

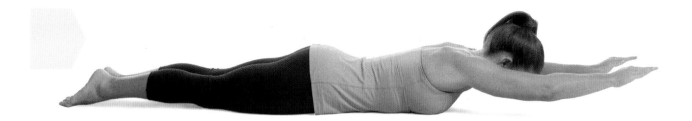

1 Lie on your stomach with your pelvis and spine in a neutral position. Extend your legs down the mat in a parallel position and hip-distance apart. At the same time, extend your arms in front of you along the mat with your palms facing down. Keep the back of your neck long with your head facing the mat. Plug your shoulders down your back.

2 Inhale, and press your navel to your spine while extending your arms into the space in front of you. Exhale.

3 Inhale, and extend legs out into the space behind your body.

4 Exhale while continuing to extend your arms and legs along your mat until they lift slightly upward.

5 Inhale and exhale in your full Superman position before releasing back down to your mat. Repeat 2 to 4 times.

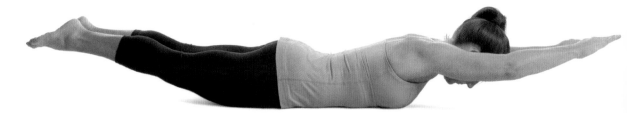

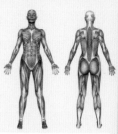

Back View

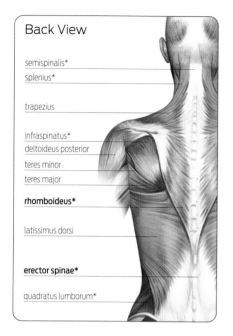

- semispinalis*
- splenius*
- trapezius
- infraspinatus*
- deltoideus posterior
- teres minor
- teres major
- **rhomboideus***
- latissimus dorsi
- **erector spinae***
- quadratus lumborum*

Front View

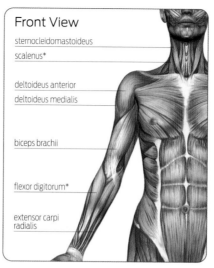

- sternocleidomastoideus
- scalenus*
- deltoideus anterior
- deltoideus medialis
- biceps brachii
- flexor digitorum*
- extensor carpi radialis

Level
- Beginner/ Intermediate

Duration
- 1–2 minutes

Benefits
- Strengthens spine and hip extensors
- Challenges stabilization of shoulder girdle
- Improves posture

Caution
- Lower-back issues
- Spinal curvature

Annotation Key
Bold text indicates target muscles
Black text indicates other working muscles
* indicates deep muscles

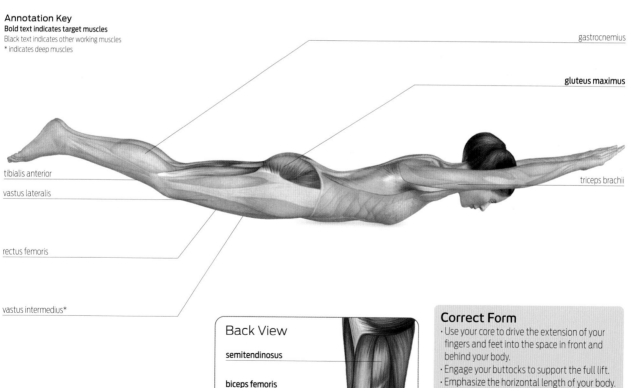

- gastrocnemius
- **gluteus maximus**
- tibialis anterior
- vastus lateralis
- triceps brachii
- rectus femoris
- vastus intermedius*

Back View

- **semitendinosus**
- **biceps femoris**
- **semimembranosus**

Correct Form
- Use your core to drive the extension of your fingers and feet into the space in front and behind your body.
- Engage your buttocks to support the full lift.
- Emphasize the horizontal length of your body.

Avoid
- Lifting your shoulders toward your ears.
- Tucking your chin into your chest.
- Arching your back.

Back Burner

In addition to strengthening your lower back, Back Burner strengthens all of your abdominal muscles. With regular practice, you'll build a sound core and improve your posture.

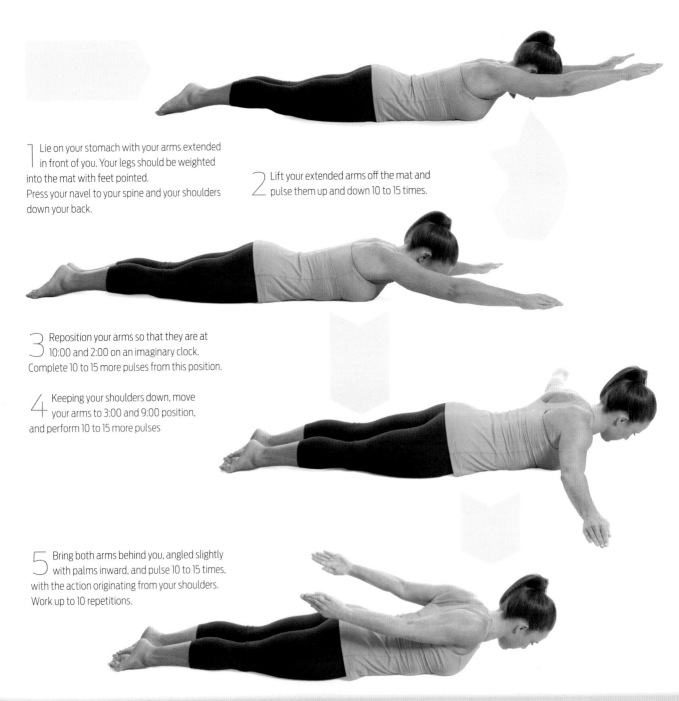

1 Lie on your stomach with your arms extended in front of you. Your legs should be weighted into the mat with feet pointed.
Press your navel to your spine and your shoulders down your back.

2 Lift your extended arms off the mat and pulse them up and down 10 to 15 times.

3 Reposition your arms so that they are at 10:00 and 2:00 on an imaginary clock. Complete 10 to 15 more pulses from this position.

4 Keeping your shoulders down, move your arms to 3:00 and 9:00 position, and perform 10 to 15 more pulses

5 Bring both arms behind you, angled slightly with palms inward, and pulse 10 to 15 times, with the action originating from your shoulders. Work up to 10 repetitions.

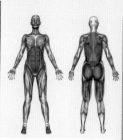

Back View

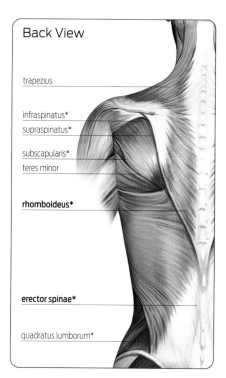

trapezius

infraspinatus*
supraspinatus*

subscapularis*
teres minor

rhomboideus*

erector spinae*

quadratus lumborum*

Front View

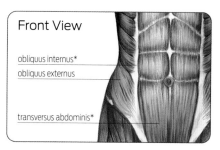

obliquus internus*
obliquus externus

transversus abdominis*

Annotation Key
Bold text indicates target muscles
Black text indicates other working muscles
* indicates deep muscles

Level
· Intermediate

Duration
· 2–3 minutes

Benefits
· Strengthens
  lower-back and
  abdominal muscles
· Improves posture

Caution ⚠
· Lower-back pain or
  other back issues
· Shoulder issues

deltoideus posterior

gluteus maximus

semitendinosus

biceps femoris

semimembranosus

Correct form
· Keep your abdominals strong and your hips stable.
· Look toward the mat to elongate your neck.
· Keep your torso and legs still throughout.
· Move your arms from under your shoulder blades.

Avoid
· Hunching your shoulders.
· Lifting your feet off the mat.

Breast Stroke

Breast Stroke adds another level of challenge to the classic Pilates Swimming exercise. It's a great stretcher and strengthener for your lower back.

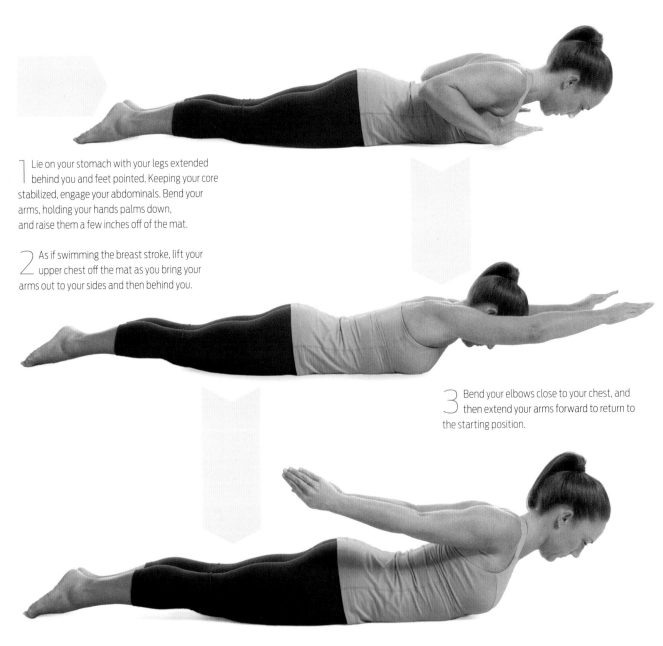

1 Lie on your stomach with your legs extended behind you and feet pointed. Keeping your core stabilized, engage your abdominals. Bend your arms, holding your hands palms down, and raise them a few inches off of the mat.

2 As if swimming the breast stroke, lift your upper chest off the mat as you bring your arms out to your sides and then behind you.

3 Bend your elbows close to your chest, and then extend your arms forward to return to the starting position.

4 Complete the entire sequence for 10 repetitions.

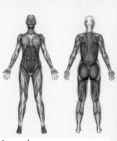

Back View

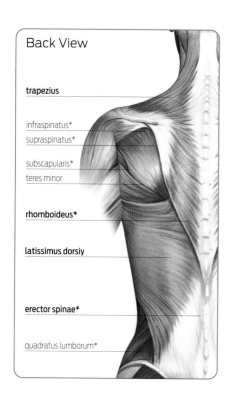

trapezius

infraspinatus*

supraspinatus*

subscapularis*

teres minor

rhomboideus*

latissimus dorsiy

erector spinae*

quadratus lumborum*

Correct form
· Keep your abdominals engaged throughout the exercise.

Avoid
· Rushing through the movement—imagine the resistance of water as you move.
· Lifting your feet off the mat.
· Hunching your shoulders to your ears.

Annotation Key
Bold text indicates target muscles
Black text indicates other working muscles
* indicates deep muscles

Level
· Intermediate/ Advanced

Duration
· 2–3 minutes

Benefits
· Strengthens upper-back muscles
· Tones core muscles

Caution
· Lower-back issues
· Shoulder issues

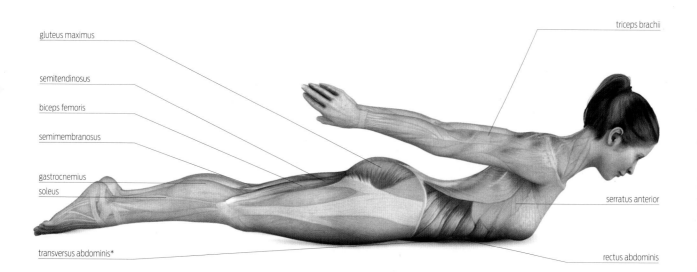

gluteus maximus

semitendinosus

biceps femoris

semimembranosus

gastrocnemius

soleus

transversus abdominis*

triceps brachii

serratus anterior

rectus abdominis

Extension Heel Beats

This exercise works your powerhouse, as well as the backs and inner parts of your legs. As with all exercises performed in a prone position, keep your abdominals fully engaged.

1 Lie on your stomach, resting your forehead on the back of your stacked hands and your elbows at shoulder height. Slightly rotate your legs from the hip joints outward and press the inner sides of your legs and your heels together. Fully engage your buttocks. Inhale to prepare.

2 Exhale as you slightly lift your extended legs up from the floor.

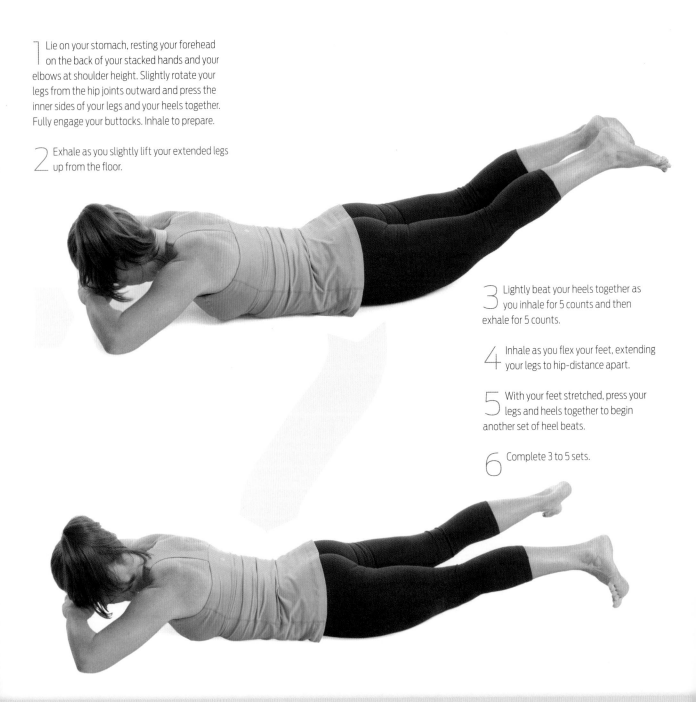

3 Lightly beat your heels together as you inhale for 5 counts and then exhale for 5 counts.

4 Inhale as you flex your feet, extending your legs to hip-distance apart.

5 With your feet stretched, press your legs and heels together to begin another set of heel beats.

6 Complete 3 to 5 sets.

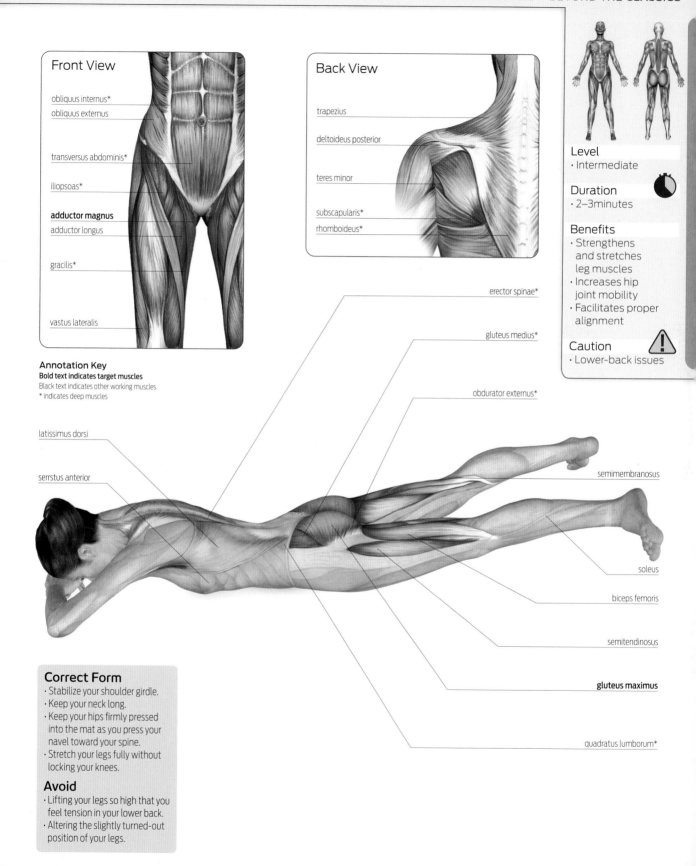

Front View

obliquus internus*
obliquus externus

transversus abdominis*

iliopsoas*

adductor magnus
adductor longus

gracilis*

vastus lateralis

Annotation Key
Bold text indicates target muscles
Black text indicates other working muscles
* indicates deep muscles

Back View

trapezius

deltoideus posterior

teres minor

subscapularis*
rhomboideus*

Level
· Intermediate

Duration
· 2–3minutes

Benefits
· Strengthens
  and stretches
  leg muscles
· Increases hip
  joint mobility
· Facilitates proper
  alignment

Caution
· Lower-back issues

erector spinae*

gluteus medius*

obdurator externus*

latissimus dorsi

serrstus anterior

semimembranosus

soleus

biceps femoris

semitendinosus

gluteus maximus

quadratus lumborum*

Correct Form
· Stabilize your shoulder girdle.
· Keep your neck long.
· Keep your hips firmly pressed
  into the mat as you press your
  navel toward your spine.
· Stretch your legs fully without
  locking your knees.

Avoid
· Lifting your legs so high that you
  feel tension in your lower back.
· Altering the slightly turned-out
  position of your legs.

Single Leg Drop

Single Leg Drop is an effective abdominal flattener. Try not to rush through the movement: it's essential that your upper body stay anchored to the mat as you lower and raise your leg—a movement driven by the strong, engaged muscles of your core.

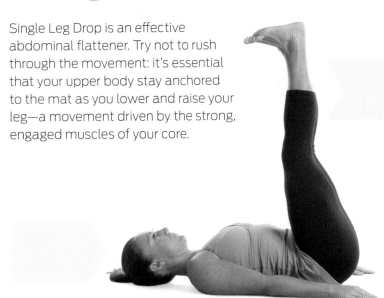

1 Lie on your back with arms at your sides and legs extended straight upward. Flex your ankles.

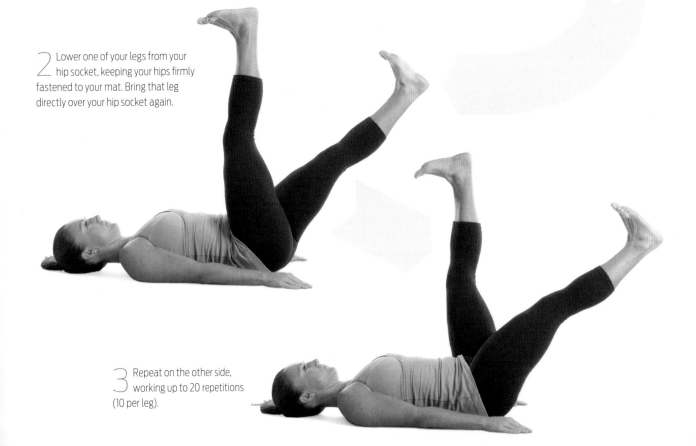

2 Lower one of your legs from your hip socket, keeping your hips firmly fastened to your mat. Bring that leg directly over your hip socket again.

3 Repeat on the other side, working up to 20 repetitions (10 per leg).

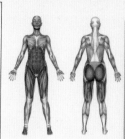

Front View

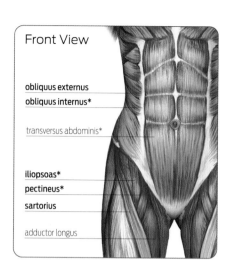

- obliquus externus
- obliquus internus*
- transversus abdominis*
- iliopsoas*
- pectineus*
- sartorius
- adductor longus

Correct form

- When your legs are extended straight up, position them directly over your hips.

Avoid

- Bringing your neck or hips off the mat.
- Arching your back.
- Using a swinging motion to lower or raise your leg. Instead, maintain steady control throughout.

Annotation Key
Bold text indicates target muscles
Black text indicates other working muscles
* indicates deep muscles

Level
- Intermediate

Duration
- 2–3 minutes

Benefits
- Tightens abs
- Strengthens core

Caution
- Lower-back issues

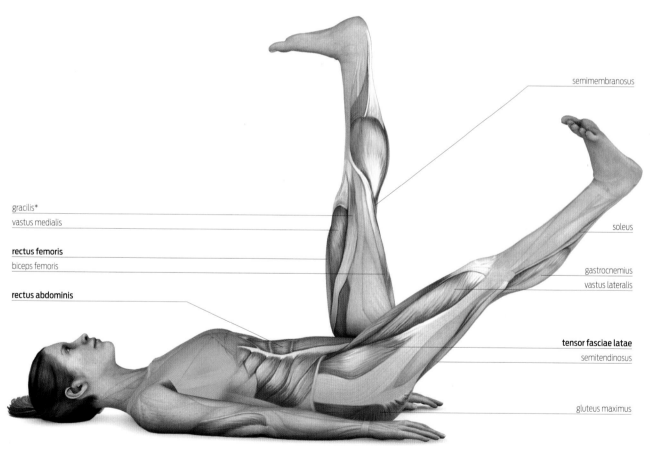

- gracilis*
- vastus medialis
- **rectus femoris**
- biceps femoris
- **rectus abdominis**

- semimembranosus
- soleus
- gastrocnemius
- vastus lateralis
- **tensor fasciae latae**
- semitendinosus
- gluteus maximus

Double Leg Drop

Double Leg Drop challenges your core muscles. The key to getting noticeable results, fast: take it slow. As your midsection stays stable and your palms press into the floor, your legs should be moving gradually and with great control.

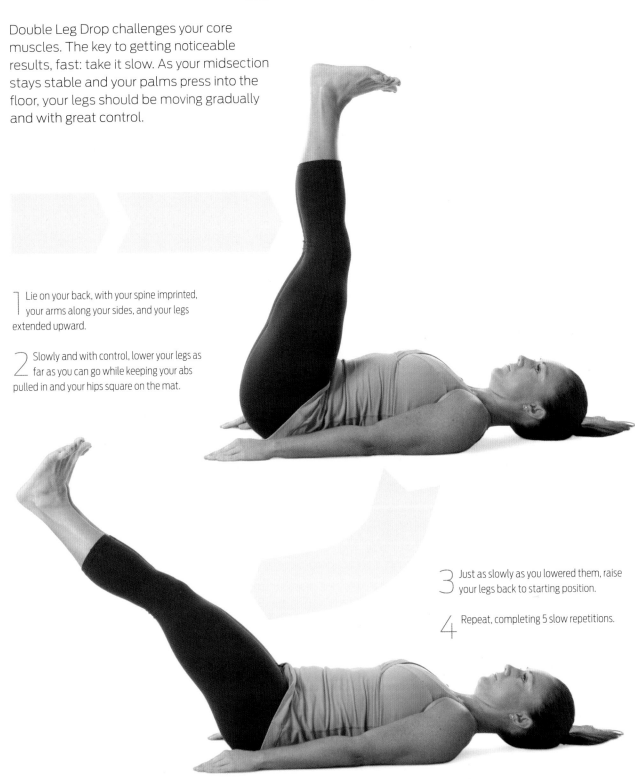

1 Lie on your back, with your spine imprinted, your arms along your sides, and your legs extended upward.

2 Slowly and with control, lower your legs as far as you can go while keeping your abs pulled in and your hips square on the mat.

3 Just as slowly as you lowered them, raise your legs back to starting position.

4 Repeat, completing 5 slow repetitions.

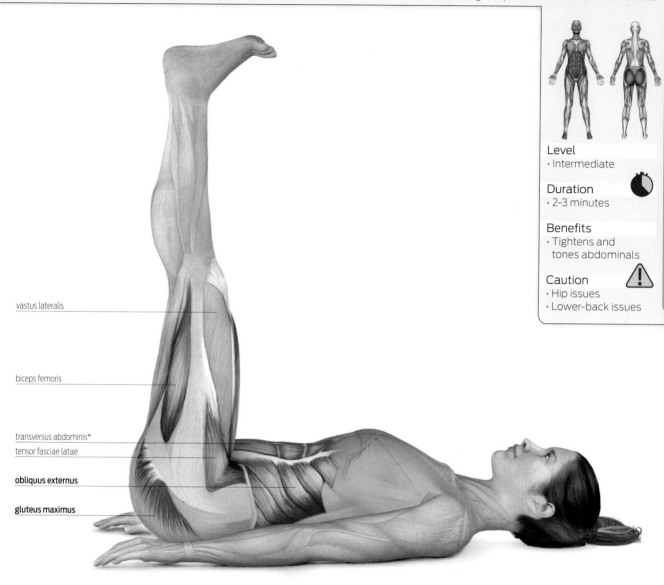

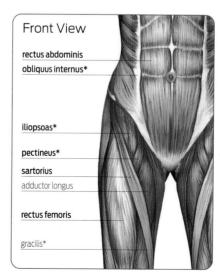

Level
· Intermediate

Duration
· 2-3 minutes

Benefits
· Tightens and
  tones abdominals

Caution
· Hip issues
· Lower-back issues

vastus lateralis

biceps femoris

transversus abdominis*

tensor fasciae latae

obliquus externus

gluteus maximus

Annotation Key
Bold text indicates target muscles
Black text indicates other working muscles
* indicates deep muscles

Correct form
· Keep your abdominals pulled in and hips
  flat on the mat.
· Move slowly and steadily.

Avoid
· Letting your lower back rise off the mat.
· Rushing through the movement.
· Lifting your neck.

Front View

rectus abdominis

obliquus internus*

iliopsoas*

pectineus*

sartorius

adductor longus

rectus femoris

gracilis*

Double Dip

Double Dip, like the Double Leg Drop works your legs and core. The ball adds extra focus on your inner-thigh muscles. Concentrate on keeping the ball perfectly still between your flexed feet. Beyond engaging your leg muscles, this will help you stay balanced and well-aligned throughout this effective, ab-flattening exercise.

1 Lie on your back, with your spine imprinted, your arms along your sides, and your legs extended upward, holding the Pilates ball between your flexed feet.

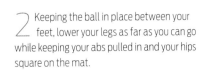

2 Keeping the ball in place between your feet, lower your legs as far as you can go while keeping your abs pulled in and your hips square on the mat.

3 Just as slowly as you lowered them, raise your legs back to starting position.

4 Repeat, performing 5 slow repetitions.

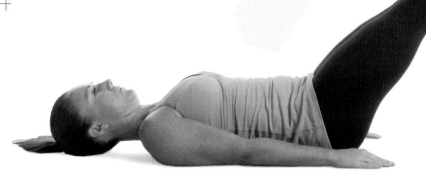

Correct form
· Keep your abdominals pulled in and hips flat on the mat.
· Move slowly and steadily.
· Focus on keeping the ball still and balanced between your feet.

Avoid
· Letting your lower back rise off the mat.
· Rushing through the movement.
· Lifting your neck.

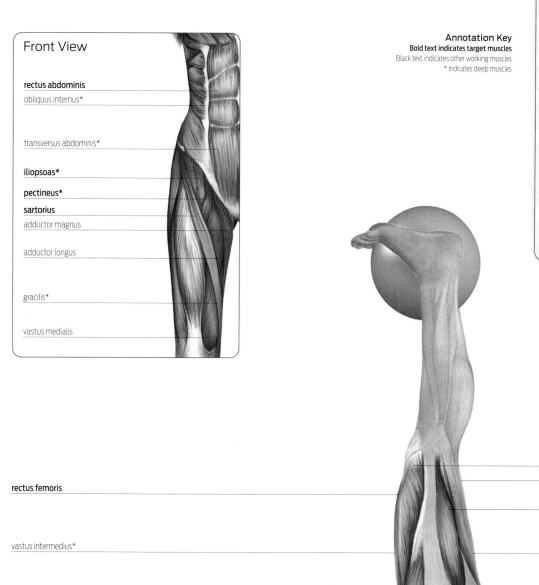

Front View

rectus abdominis

obliquus internus*

transversus abdominis*

iliopsoas*

pectineus*

sartorius

adductor magnus

adductor longus

gracilis*

vastus medialis

Annotation Key
Bold text indicates target muscles
Black text indicates other working muscles
* indicates deep muscles

Level
· Intermediate

Duration
· 2–3 minutes

Benefits
· Tightens and tones abdominals
· Strengthens and tones leg muscles

Caution ⚠
· Hip issues
· Lower-back issues

rectus femoris

vastus intermedius*

vastus lateralis

semimembranosus

biceps femoris

semitendinosus

tensor fasciae latae

obliquus externus

gluteus maximus

Basic Crunch

Basic Crunch, also called Curl-Up, is a popular abdominal exercise. To perform it the Pilates way, think centering, control, flow, breath, precision, and concentration. When your pelvis is in neutral, you should be able to slide a hand under your lumbar spine.

Correct Form
- Use your abdominals to initiate the curl.
- Hold your legs firmly together, engaging your inner thighs and buttocks.
- Keep your elbows wide.

Avoid
- Lifting your chin, or tucking it into your chest.
- Tucking your pelvis.

1 Lie on your back with your spine and pelvis in a neutral position, your legs bent and parallel, your feet planted on your mat, and your toes spread and relaxed.

2 Place your hands, stacked one on top of the other, behind your head—with your elbows wide. Inhale to prepare.

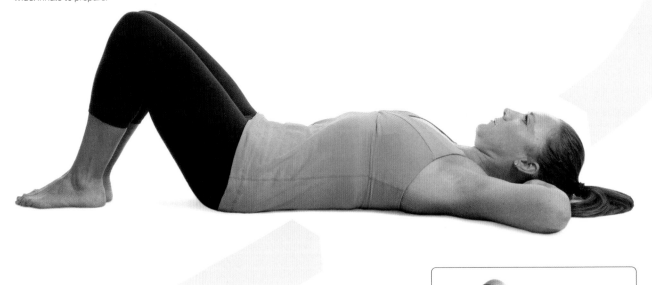

Modification
Harder: Place a ball between your knees to add lower body resistance to the exercise. This modification activates your inner thighs and buttocks and provides you with a physical cue as to how to activate your legs when you don't have the ball.

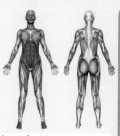

3 Exhale and curl up to the lower tip of your shoulder blades, looking diagonally forward.

5 Repeat 6 to 10 times.

4 Inhale as you roll down to your mat again.

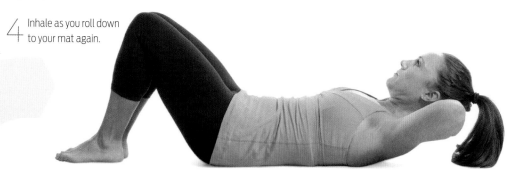

Level
· Beginner

Duration
· 1–2 minutes

Benefits
· Strengthens torso
· Improves pelvic and core stability

Caution
· Back pain
· Neck issues

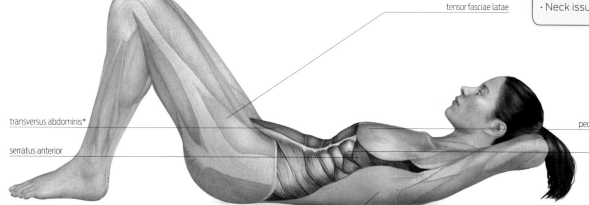

tensor fasciae latae

transversus abdominis*

serratus anterior

pectoralis major

obliquus externus

latissimus dorsi

Front View

sternocleidomastoideus

scalenus*

deltoideus anterior

pectoralis minor*

coracobrachialis*

biceps brachii

rectus abdominis

iliopsoas*

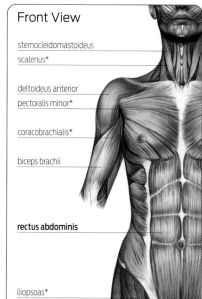

Back View

splenius*

trapezius

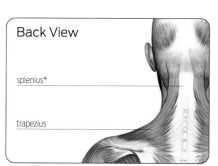

Annotation Key
Bold text indicates target muscles
Black text indicates other working muscles
* indicates deep muscles

Figure 8

The challenge of this exercise is to maintain your spinal c-curve, with its accompanying abdominal support, while engaging your upper back in a figure 8–like motion: not so easy, though great for maximizing the power of your powerhouse.

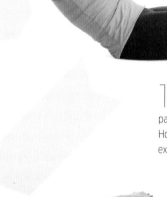

1 Start by sitting tall on top of your hipbones, with your knees bent, pressed together and parallel, and your feet firmly planted into your mat. Hold your ball between your hands with your arms extended in front of you. Inhale to prepare.

2 Exhale as you press your navel toward your spine. Imprint your pelvis as you straighten your legs along the mat. Roll back to about 45 degrees, controlling your abdominals as you press your legs firmly down into your mat.

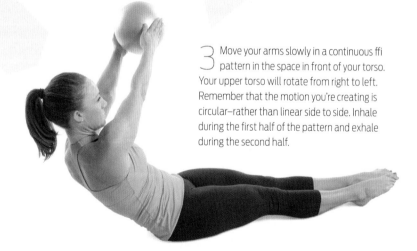

3 Move your arms slowly in a continuous ffi pattern in the space in front of your torso. Your upper torso will rotate from right to left. Remember that the motion you're creating is circular–rather than linear side to side. Inhale during the first half of the pattern and exhale during the second half.

Correct Form
· Use your abdominals to initiate the movement.
· Keep your shoulders blades pressed down your back.
· Keep your legs pressed tightly together.

Avoid
· Lifting your chin toward the ceiling.
· Lifting your feet off your mat.
· Changing the position of your spine.
· Holding your breath.

Figure 8 • BEYOND THE CLASSICS

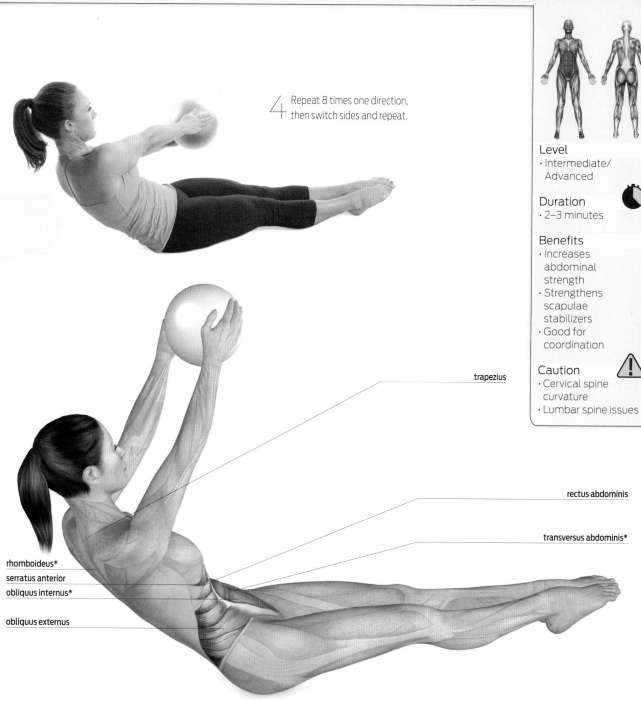

4 Repeat 8 times one direction, then switch sides and repeat.

Level
· Intermediate/ Advanced

Duration
· 2–3 minutes

Benefits
· Increases abdominal strength
· Strengthens scapulae stabilizers
· Good for coordination

Caution
· Cervical spine curvature
· Lumbar spine issues

trapezius

rectus abdominis

transversus abdominis*

rhomboideus*

serratus anterior

obliquus internus*

obliquus externus

Annotation Key
Bold text indicates target muscles
Black text indicates other working muscles
* indicates deep muscles

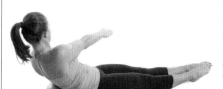

Modification

Try doing Figure 8 with your ball placed at the small of your back for support, rather than between your hands. This easier version allows you to focus on the upper body coordination without compromising the correct position of your spine and pelvis.

C-Curve Arm Cross

This exercise uses the same position as the Figure 8 modification exercise (page 109). You have to maintain that powerful c-curve connection between the front and back of your torso, and work your arms between your shoulder blades: a good exercise in multitasking! You can always add small hand weights for greater upper-body resistance.

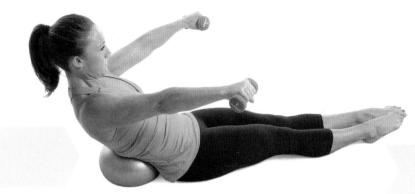

1 Start by sitting tall on top of your hipbones, with your parallel legs, bent and pressed together, and your feet firmly planted into your mat. Have the ball by your side, ready for use. Extend your arms in front of you, parallel to your knees. Inhale to prepare.

2 Exhale as you press your navel toward your spine. Imprint your pelvis and straighten your legs along the mat. Roll back to about 45 degrees, maintaining strong abdominals and pressing your legs firmly together. Place the ball behind your back so it comfortably supports your lumbar spine.

3 With your palms facing down toward the floor, cross your right arm over the left and then the left arm over the right in quick–though controlled– movements. Exhale for 5 arm beats and inhale for 5 arm beats.

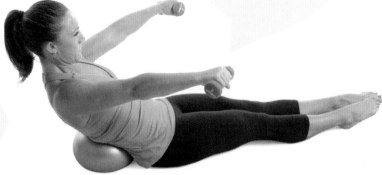

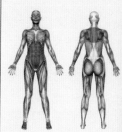

4 Cross your arms 10 times, which equals 1 set. Try to build up to 10 sets.

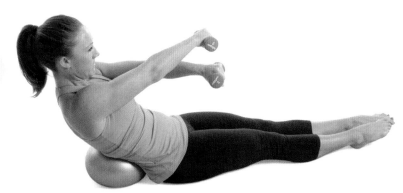

Level
· Intermediate/ Advanced

Duration
· 3–4 minutes

Benefits
· Stabilizes shoulder girdle
· Strengthens upper body
· Increases abdominal strength.

Caution
· Lumbar spine issues
· Cervical spine curvature
· Severe neck tension

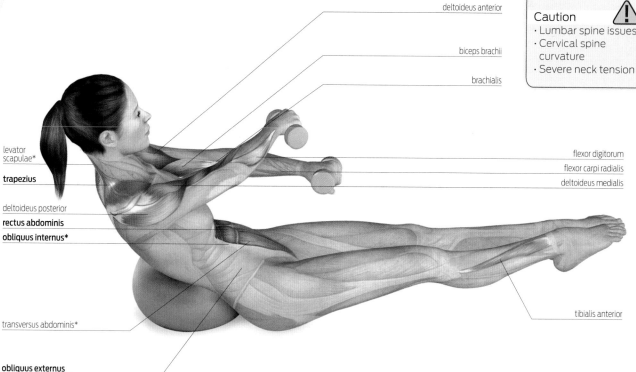

deltoideus anterior

biceps brachii

brachialis

levator scapulae*

trapezius

deltoideus posterior

rectus abdominis

obliquus internus*

transversus abdominis*

obliquus externus

flexor digitorum

flexor carpi radialis

deltoideus medialis

tibialis anterior

Annotation Key
Bold text indicates target muscles
Black text indicates other working muscles
* indicates deep muscles

Correct Form.
· Keep your arm movements steady and controlled.
· Keep your shoulders blades pressed down your back.
· Use your inner thighs to keep your legs firmly planted.

Avoid
· Lifting your chin toward the ceiling.
· Lifting your feet from your mat.
· Altering the imprinted position of your pelvis.
· Locking your elbows or knees.

Pilates Ball Tabletop Bridge

Pilates Ball Tabletop Bridge targets your buttocks, thighs, shoulders, and abdominals. Challenge yourself to maintain one long, straight, line from your shoulders to knees while in the bridge position. Really use that ball, and you'll feel your body getting stronger and more toned.

1 Lie on your back with your arms along your sides and your legs in tabletop position with the Pilates ball between your knees.

2 Lower your feet to the mat, using your abdominals to drive the movement.

3 Press your arms into the mat for stability, engage your buttocks, and lift your pelvis so that your body from shoulders to legs forms a bridge. Use your inner-thigh muscles to hold the ball in place.

4 Stay in the bridge for a few seconds before relaxing your spine down to the mat and then returning to the tabletop position again.

5 Complete 5 repetitions.

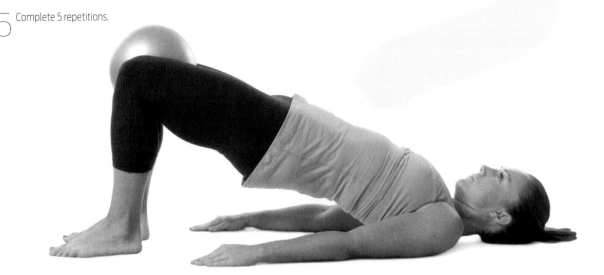

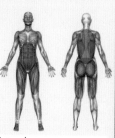

Annotation Key
Bold text indicates target muscles
Black text indicates other working muscles
* indicates deep muscles

Correct form
· Keep your navel pressed toward your spine.
· Engage your buttocks, thighs, and hamstrings.
· Keep your pelvis level while in the bridge.

Avoid
· Allowing your hips to sink toward the mat.
· Arching your back while in the bridge.

Level
· Intermediate

Duration
· 2–3 minutes

Benefits
· Increases stability in pelvis and spine
· Improves hip flexor endurance

Caution
· Neck issues
· Severe knee injury

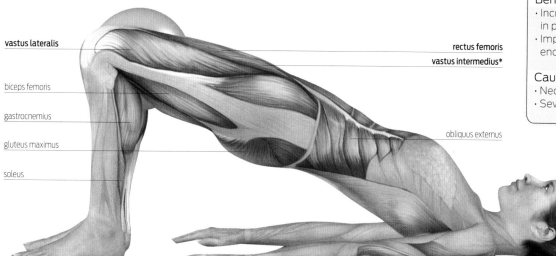

vastus lateralis

biceps femoris

gastrocnemius

gluteus maximus

soleus

rectus femoris

vastus intermedius*

obliquus externus

triceps brachii

deltoideus medialis

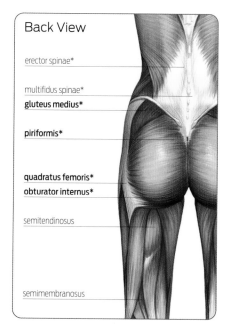

Back View

erector spinae*

multifidus spinae*

gluteus medius*

piriformis*

quadratus femoris*

obturator internus*

semitendinosus

semimembranosus

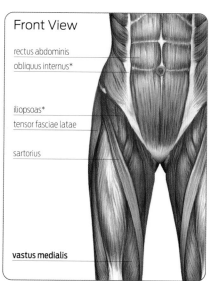

Front View

rectus abdominis

obliquus internus*

iliopsoas*

tensor fasciae latae

sartorius

vastus medialis

Tabletop March

Tabletop March stretches the entire front of your body while strengthening your supporting back and legs. Try this exercise as a continuation of the Shoulder Bridge exercise (see pages 54–55). When you add the march to the bridge, you'll work your legs from your hip joints.

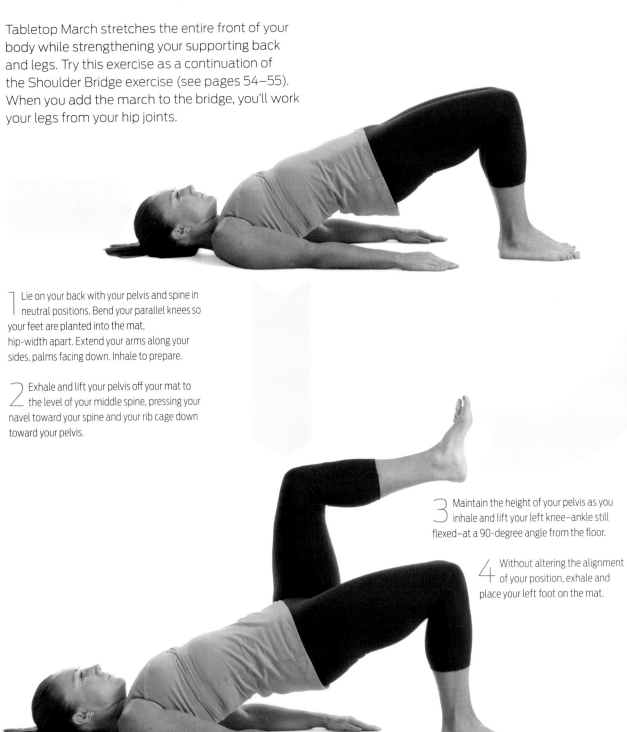

1 Lie on your back with your pelvis and spine in neutral positions. Bend your parallel knees so your feet are planted into the mat, hip-width apart. Extend your arms along your sides, palms facing down. Inhale to prepare.

2 Exhale and lift your pelvis off your mat to the level of your middle spine, pressing your navel toward your spine and your rib cage down toward your pelvis.

3 Maintain the height of your pelvis as you inhale and lift your left knee–ankle still flexed–at a 90-degree angle from the floor.

4 Without altering the alignment of your position, exhale and place your left foot on the mat.

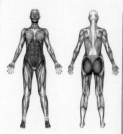

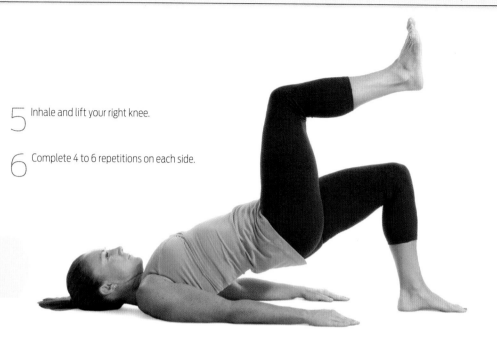

5 Inhale and lift your right knee.

6 Complete 4 to 6 repetitions on each side.

Level
· Intermediate

Duration
· 2–4 minutes

Benefits
· Strengthens hip extensors.
· Improves shoulder and hip stabilization.
· Works single-leg balance.

Caution ⚠
· Severe knee issues

Correct Form
· Maintain your neutral spine alignment throughout.
· Keep your neck long with your chin pointed slightly toward your chest.
· Keep the leg on the mat in a strong parallel position.

Avoid
· Pinching the vertebrae of your neck.
· Shifting the height of your hips.
· Pressing into your lumbar spine.

Annotation Key
Bold text indicates target muscles
Black text indicates other working muscles
* indicates deep muscles

sartorius
adductor longus
adductor brevis
adductor magnus
pectineus*
iliopsoas*
transversus abdominis*
rectus abdominis

vastus medialis
vastus lateralis
rectus femoris
vastus intermedius*
biceps femoris
obliquus internus*
obliquus externus
gluteus medius*
gluteus maximus

High Bridge Leg Drops

After doing the Shoulder Bridge you could continue with Tabletop March or this exercise, High Bridge Leg Drops. This is an advanced exercise, since it requires a strong and stable core, solid powerhouse control, and stamina.

1 Lie on your back with your pelvis and spine in neutral. Bend your parallel knees so your feet are planted into the mat, hip-width apart. Extend your arms along your sides, palms facing down. Inhale to prepare.

2 Exhale and lift your pelvis off your mat to the level of your middle spine, pressing your navel toward your spine and your rib cage down toward your pelvis.

3 Maintain your bridge position as you inhale and extend your right leg so that it's level with your left knee.

4 Exhale and raise your right leg toward the ceiling, directly over your right hip joint.

5 Inhale and lower your right leg so that it's level with your left knee.

Correct Form
· Maintain your neutral spine throughout.
· Press the whole supporting foot down into the mat.
· Maintain the precise angular shape of your free leg.

Avoid
· Rotating your hips.
· Pinching the vertebrae in your neck.
· "Popping" your rib cage or your abdominals

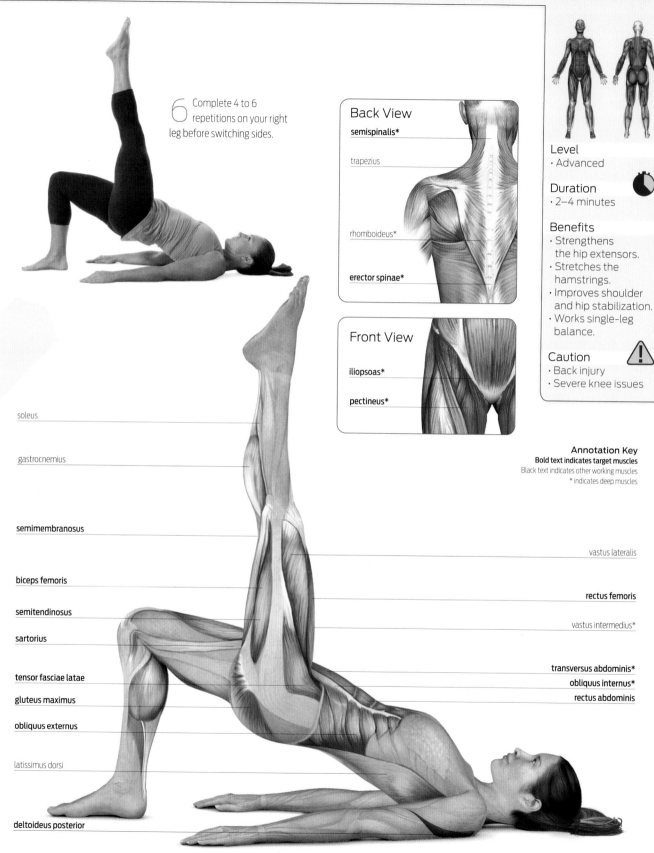

6 Complete 4 to 6 repetitions on your right leg before switching sides.

Back View

semispinalis*

trapezius

rhomboideus*

erector spinae*

Front View

iliopsoas*

pectineus*

Level
· Advanced

Duration
· 2–4 minutes

Benefits
· Strengthens the hip extensors.
· Stretches the hamstrings.
· Improves shoulder and hip stabilization.
· Works single-leg balance.

Caution
· Back injury
· Severe knee issues

Annotation Key
Bold text indicates target muscles
Black text indicates other working muscles
* indicates deep muscles

soleus

gastrocnemius

semimembranosus

biceps femoris

semitendinosus

sartorius

tensor fasciae latae

gluteus maximus

obliquus externus

latissimus dorsi

deltoideus posterior

vastus lateralis

rectus femoris

vastus intermedius*

transversus abdominis*

obliquus internus*

rectus abdominis

Waistline Warrior

Waistline Warrior may look simple
enough, but these small movements
really challenge your oblique muscles.

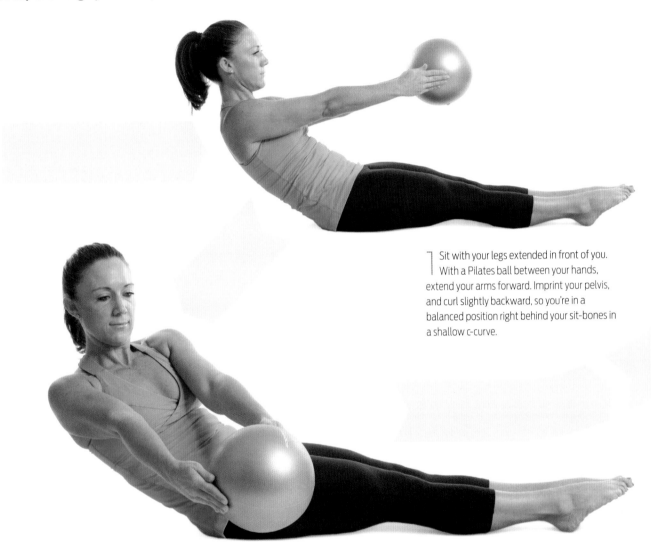

1 Sit with your legs extended in front of you.
With a Pilates ball between your hands,
extend your arms forward. Imprint your pelvis,
and curl slightly backward, so you're in a
balanced position right behind your sit-bones in
a shallow c-curve.

2 Keeping your abdominals tight and your
legs firmly on the mat, squeeze your inner
thighs and rotate your torso slightly to the right,
bringing the ball with you.

Correct form
· Curl back only as far as you can maintain
  control of your abdominals and legs.
· Follow the ball with your gaze.
· Hold your arms in a slightly curved shape.

Avoid
· Lifting your legs off the mat.
· Rushing through the movement; your pace
  should be smooth, steady, and controlled.

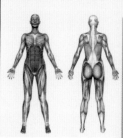

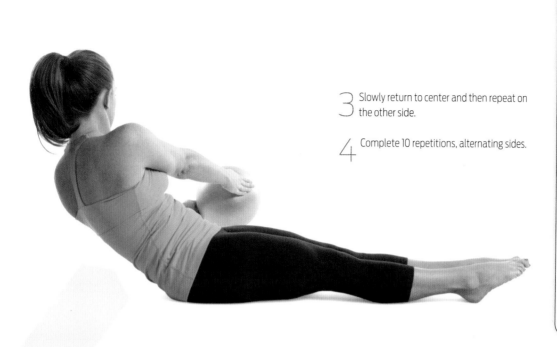

3 Slowly return to center and then repeat on the other side.

4 Complete 10 repetitions, alternating sides.

Level
· Intermediate

Duration
· 2–3 minutes

Benefits
· Tones and tightens obliques
· Stabilizes core

Caution
· Neck issues
· Lower-back pain or other back issues

Annotation Key
Bold text indicates target muscles
Black text indicates other working muscles
* indicates deep muscles

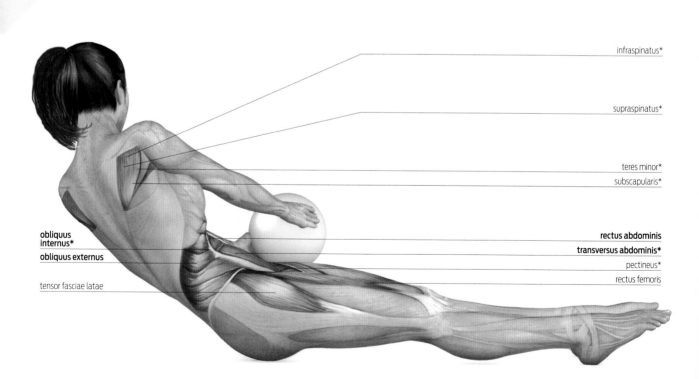

infraspinatus*

supraspinatus*

teres minor*
subscapularis*

obliquus internus*
obliquus externus

tensor fasciae latae

rectus abdominis
transversus abdominis*
pectineus*
rectus femoris

Bicycle Twist

When executing Bicycle Twists with good form, you'll get the satisfying sense that your abdominals are working hard—and getting harder in the process. Especially beneficial to the hard-to-reach obliques, these twists can be fast-paced; be sure to stay mindful of your core, engaging your abdominals throughout the entire sequence.

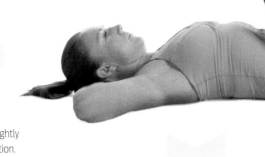

1 Lie on your back, with your knees bent slightly closer to your body than in tabletop position. Place your hands behind your head, and raise your upper body off the mat.

2 Extend one leg downward as far as you can go while keeping your pelvis stable and abdominals pulled in. At the same time, bring the other knee toward your chest and rotate your upper body diagonally so that your knee touches the opposite elbow.

Correct form
· Touch your elbow to your opposite knee with each twist.
· Return to starting position between every twist.
· Keep your elbows wide.
· Maintain pointed feet throughout the exercise.

Avoid
· Holding your breath.
· Pushing your head with your hands; instead, the lifting of your upper body should come from your core, particularly your obliques.
· Letting your abdominals bulge outward.
· Hunching your shoulders.
· Lowering your leg so far that you arch your back.

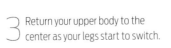

3 Return your upper body to the center as your legs start to switch.

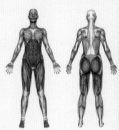

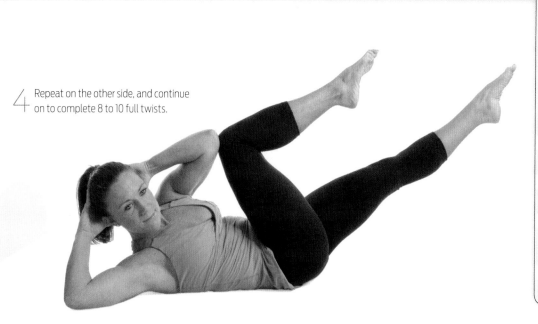

4 Repeat on the other side, and continue on to complete 8 to 10 full twists.

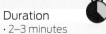

Level
· Intermediate

Duration
· 2–3 minutes

Benefits
· Strengthens and tones abdominals

Caution
· Neck pain

Annotation Key
Bold text indicates target muscles
Black text indicates other working muscles
* indicates deep muscles

Front View
rectus abdominis
obliquus internus*
transversus abdominis*

iliopsoas*
pectineus*

vastus intermedius*

rectus femoris
vastus medialis

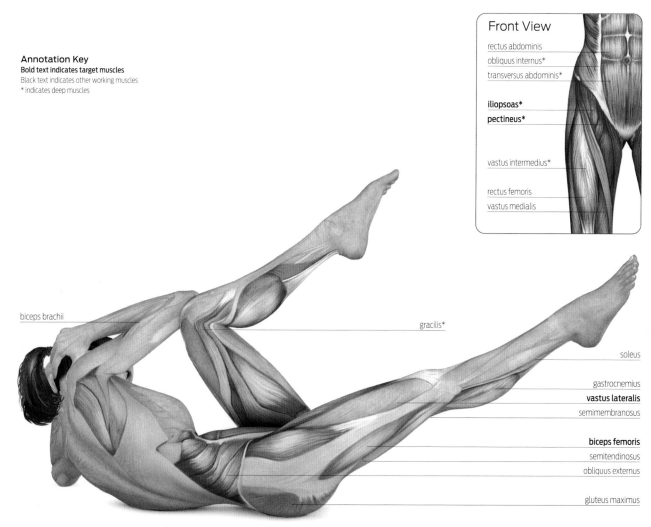

biceps brachii

gracilis*

soleus

gastrocnemius
vastus lateralis
semimembranosus

biceps femoris
semitendinosus
obliquus externus

gluteus maximus

Criss-Cross

Criss-Cross strengthens your abdominals, enhances the stability of your torso, and stretches and tones your legs. Be prepared to coordinate core control with the flowing rhythmic movements of your legs.

Modification

Easier: Perform the exercise with your knees bent. Keep your legs close together during the crisscross so that your inner thighs brush each other. Stretching through the arches of your feet helps to keep your legs fully engaged.

1 Lie on your back with your arms by your sides and your legs extended up in the air above your hip joints. Imprint your pelvis and anchor your core firmly to the mat. Both sides of your neck should be long and your throat free of tension. To gain greater control over your leg movements, rotate your legs slightly in the hips. Inhale to prepare.

2 Exhale as you cross your ankles forward and back of each other while lowering your legs toward the mat.

Correct Form
· Roll your shoulders back and down your spine.
· Work in a small range initially, until strength and stamina have developed.
· Use your inner thighs, as well as your buttock muscles, to control the flow of the legs.

Avoid
· Allowing your back to arch off the mat as you lower your legs.
· Rounding your shoulders forward.
· Relaxing your feet.

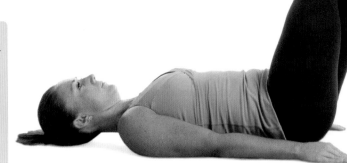

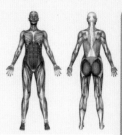

3 Inhale while raising your legs to vertical again, crisscrossing your ankles all the way up.

4 Complete 10 to 20 sets.

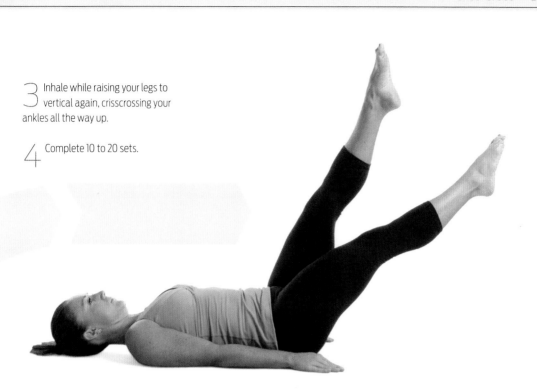

Level
· Intermediate/ Advanced

Duration
· 2–3 minutes

Benefits
· Facilitates hip mobility
· Promotes core stability and strength

Caution
· Cervical or lumbar spine curvature
· Hip injury or surgery
· Lower-back issues

Front View

rectus abdominis

transversus abdominis*

iliopsoas*

pectineus*

adductor magnus

adductor longus

Annotation Key
Bold text indicates target muscles
Black text indicates other working muscles
* indicates deep muscles

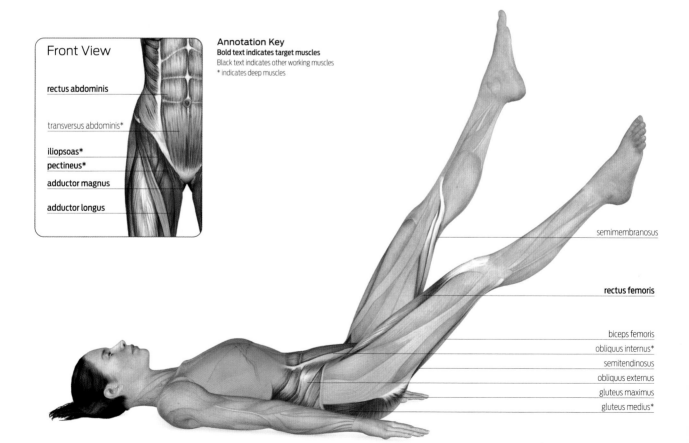

semimembranosus

rectus femoris

biceps femoris

obliquus internus*

semitendinosus

obliquus externus

gluteus maximus

gluteus medius*

Single-Leg Heel Taps

Although seemingly simple, Single-Leg Heel Taps offers beginners—as well as advanced practitioners—the chance to concentrate on the basic Pilates principles of centering, control, flow, breath, precision, and concentration.

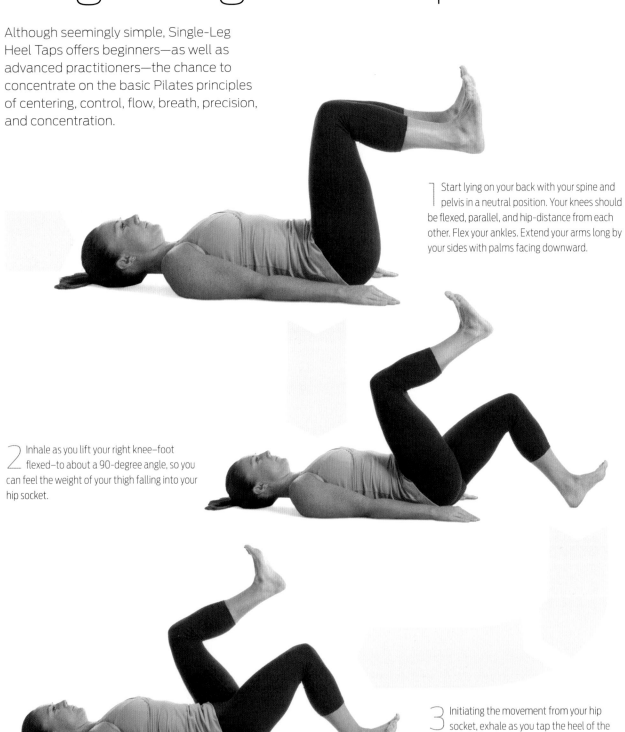

1 Start lying on your back with your spine and pelvis in a neutral position. Your knees should be flexed, parallel, and hip-distance from each other. Flex your ankles. Extend your arms long by your sides with palms facing downward.

2 Inhale as you lift your right knee—foot flexed—to about a 90-degree angle, so you can feel the weight of your thigh falling into your hip socket.

3 Initiating the movement from your hip socket, exhale as you tap the heel of the right foot to the floor. Change to your left leg. Repeat 6 to 10 times, alternating legs.

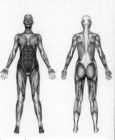

Annotation Key
Bold text indicates target muscles
Black text indicates other working muscles
* indicates deep muscles

Correct Form
· Stabilized your torso throughout.
· Keep your knees parallel.
· Keep your tapping heel in line with the supporting heel.
· Flex your ankles and put weight onto your heels.

Avoid
· Lifting your chin toward the ceiling.
· Losing the neutral position of your spine or pelvis.

Level
· Beginner

Duration
· 1–2 minutes

Benefits
· Increases core stability
· Increases mobility in hip joints
· Improves posture

Caution
· Neck strain

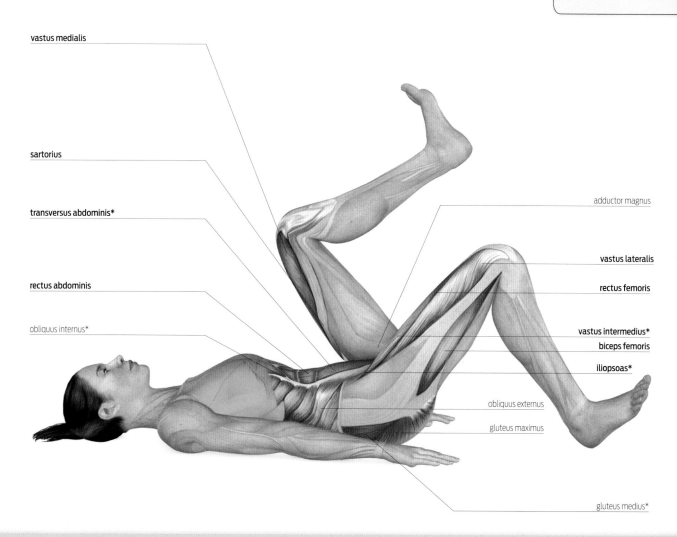

vastus medialis

sartorius

transversus abdominis*

rectus abdominis

obliquus internus*

adductor magnus

vastus lateralis

rectus femoris

vastus intermedius*

biceps femoris

iliopsoas*

obliquus externus

gluteus maximus

gluteus medius*

Pilates Ball Heel Taps

This version of Heel Tap improves your core stability and strength, enhancing your alignment and flattening your abdominals in the process. With the Pilates ball between your knees, your inner thighs get a great workout too.

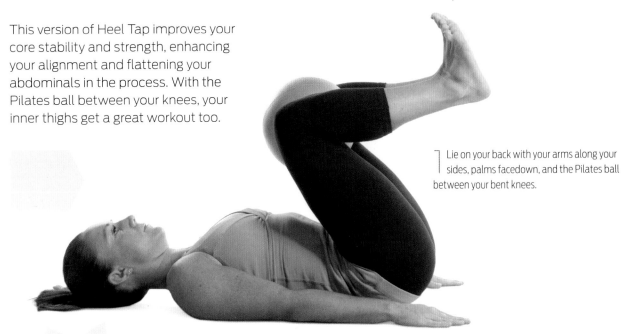

1 Lie on your back with your arms along your sides, palms facedown, and the Pilates ball between your bent knees.

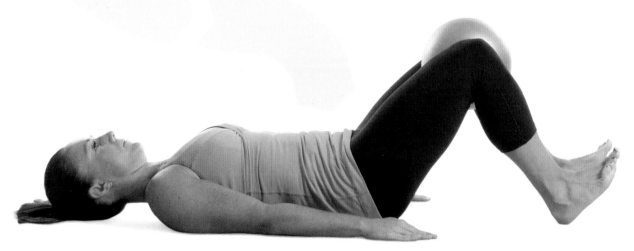

2 Keeping your upper body anchored on your mat, press your navel to your spine and dip your heels down toward your mat, hugging your inner thighs around the Pilates ball. Tap your heels to the mat.

3 Bring your legs back into your chest as you return to starting position.

4 Complete 10 repetitions.

Correct form
· Keep your abdominals strongly connected to your lower spine and your pelvis in imprint.

Avoid
· Arching your cervical or lumbar spine.

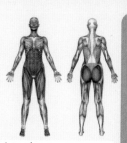

Front View

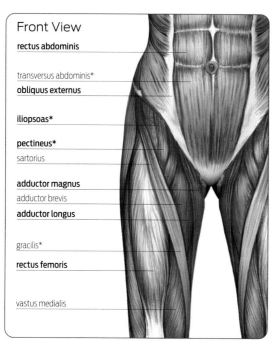

rectus abdominis

transversus abdominis*
obliquus externus

iliopsoas*

pectineus*
sartorius

adductor magnus
adductor brevis
adductor longus

gracilis*
rectus femoris

vastus medialis

Annotation Key
Bold text indicates target muscles
Black text indicates other working muscles
* indicates deep muscles

Level
· Intermediate

Duration
· 2–3 minutes

Benefits
· Improves core strength and stability
· Tightens and tones abdominal muscles

Caution
· Lower-back issues

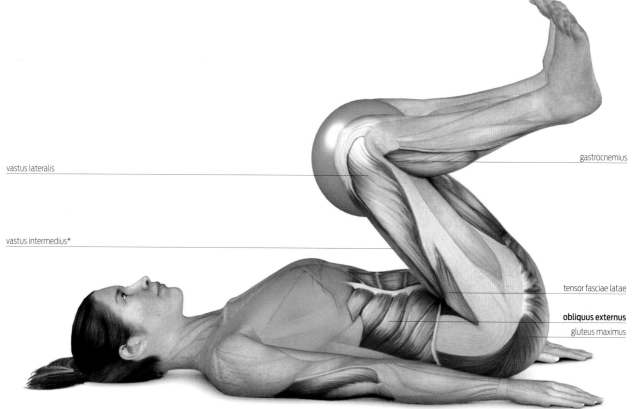

vastus lateralis

vastus intermedius*

gastrocnemius

tensor fasciae latae

obliquus externus
gluteus maximus

Double-Leg Heel Taps

Double-Leg Heel Taps offer a more challenging variation on Single-Leg Heel Taps. You have both legs off the floor at the same time, which requires greater integrated work between your abdominals and back. Remember, too, that the neutral spine is used with exercises where one or two legs are on the mat. In Double-Leg Heel Taps you'll have both legs off your mat, which means that you'll be working from an imprint position.

1 As with Single-Leg Heel Taps, lie on your back. Your knees should be flexed, parallel, and hip-distance from each other, your ankles flexed, and your arms extended along your sides with palms facing upward. This time, imprint your spine and pelvis.

2 Inhale as you lift your knees, aiming to form about a 90-degree angle with your mat so that you can feel the weight of your thighs falling into your hip sockets.

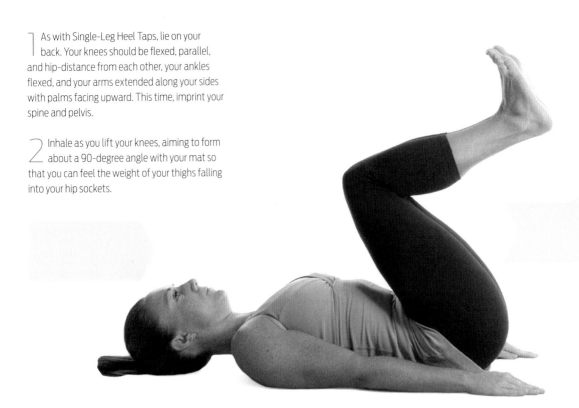

Correct Form
· Maintain your stabilized torso throughout.
· Keep your knees flexed as you lift your knees.
· Keep your knees parallel and positioned hip-width apart.
· Flex your ankles strongly as if you were pressing against a wall.

Avoid
· Forgetting to imprint.
· Losing the length along the sides of your neck.
· Allowing your rib cage or stomach muscles to pop up.

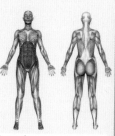

3 Initiating the movement from your hip sockets, exhale while tapping the heels of your feet to your mat.

4 Repeat 8 to 12 times.

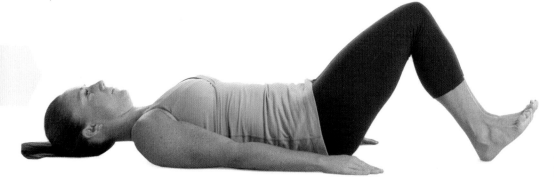

Level
· Intermediate

Duration
· 2–3 minutes

Benefits
· Increases core stability
· Improves shoulder girdle stability
· Strengthens abdominals
· Provides awareness of the leg-pelvis dynamic

Caution
· Hip tightness
· Neck strain
· Spinal injury

Front View

transversus abdominis*

iliopsoas*
pectineus*
sartorius
adductor magnus
adductor brevis
adductor longus

gracilis*
rectus femoris

vastus medialis

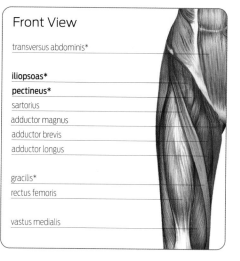

Annotation Key
Bold text indicates target muscles
Black text indicates other working muscles
* indicates deep muscles

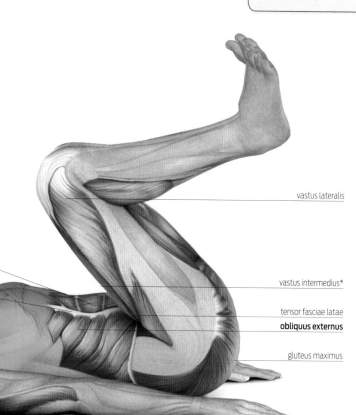

vastus lateralis

rectus abdominis

obliquus internus*

vastus intermedius*

tensor fasciae latae
obliquus externus

gluteus maximus

Frog

Frog will really target your hip flexors and extensors—working your buttocks and abdominals along the way.

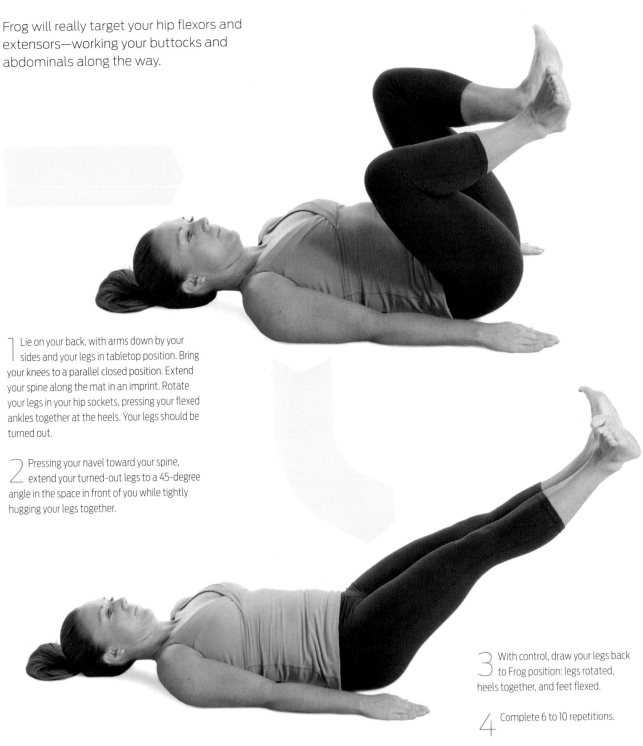

1 Lie on your back, with arms down by your sides and your legs in tabletop position. Bring your knees to a parallel closed position. Extend your spine along the mat in an imprint. Rotate your legs in your hip sockets, pressing your flexed ankles together at the heels. Your legs should be turned out.

2 Pressing your navel toward your spine, extend your turned-out legs to a 45-degree angle in the space in front of you while tightly hugging your legs together.

3 With control, draw your legs back to Frog position: legs rotated, heels together, and feet flexed.

4 Complete 6 to 10 repetitions.

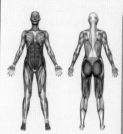

Front View

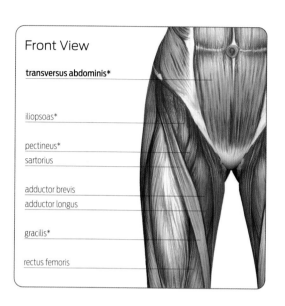

transversus abdominis*

iliopsoas*

pectineus*

sartorius

adductor brevis

adductor longus

gracilis*

rectus femoris

Annotation Key
Bold text indicates target muscles
Black text indicates other working muscles
* indicates deep muscles

Correct form
· Rotate your legs from your hip sockets.

Avoid
· Lowering your legs too far; go only as low as you can maintain complete control.
· Arching your back.
· Dropping your heels toward the mat when bringing your knees in.

Level
· Intermediate

Duration
· 2–3 minutes

Benefits
· Strengthens and tones abdominals and glutes
· Strengthens hip flexors and extensors

Caution
· Hip issues
· Lower-back pain or other back issues

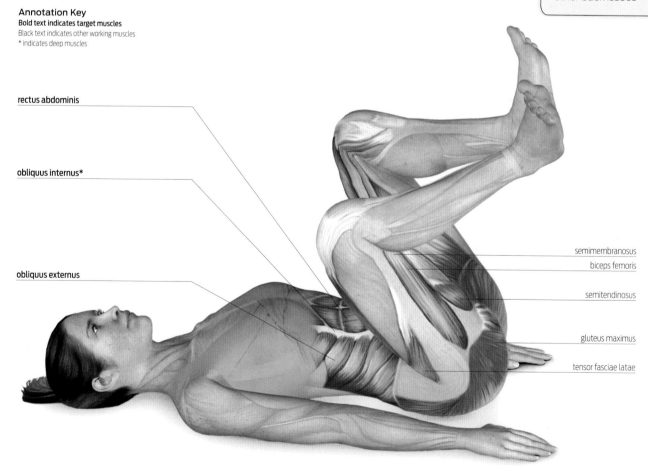

rectus abdominis

obliquus internus*

obliquus externus

semimembranosus

biceps femoris

semitendinosus

gluteus maximus

tensor fasciae latae

Single-Leg Gluteal Lift

Pilates may be known for developing sleek and strong abdominals, but the Single-Leg Gluteal Lift proves that it develops tight buttocks too. When lifting, raise your body only as high as you can go while maintaining correct alignment. If you feel strain in your lower back, you're going too far.

1 Lie on your back with your arms along your sides and legs bent with your feet directly under your knees. Extend one leg upward, pointing through your foot.

2 Engage your abdominals to pop up to a one-legged, stable bridge.

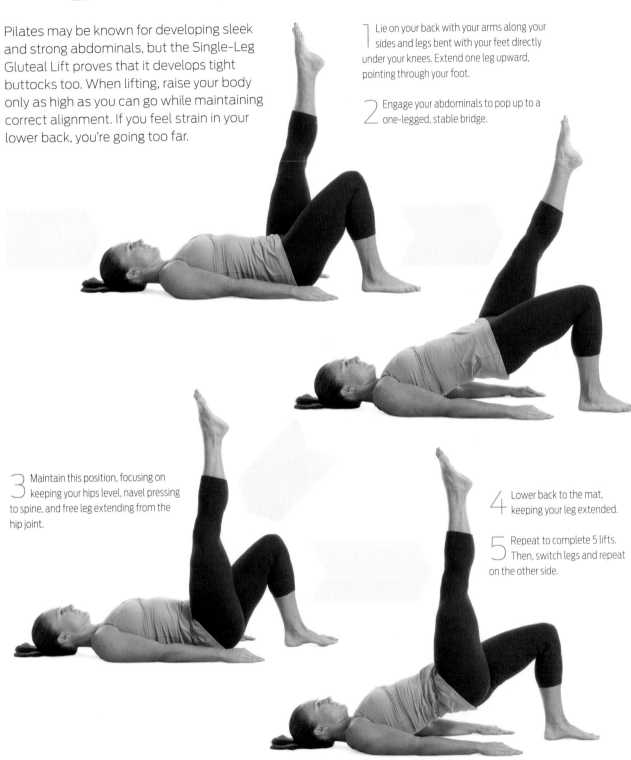

3 Maintain this position, focusing on keeping your hips level, navel pressing to spine, and free leg extending from the hip joint.

4 Lower back to the mat, keeping your leg extended.

5 Repeat to complete 5 lifts. Then, switch legs and repeat on the other side.

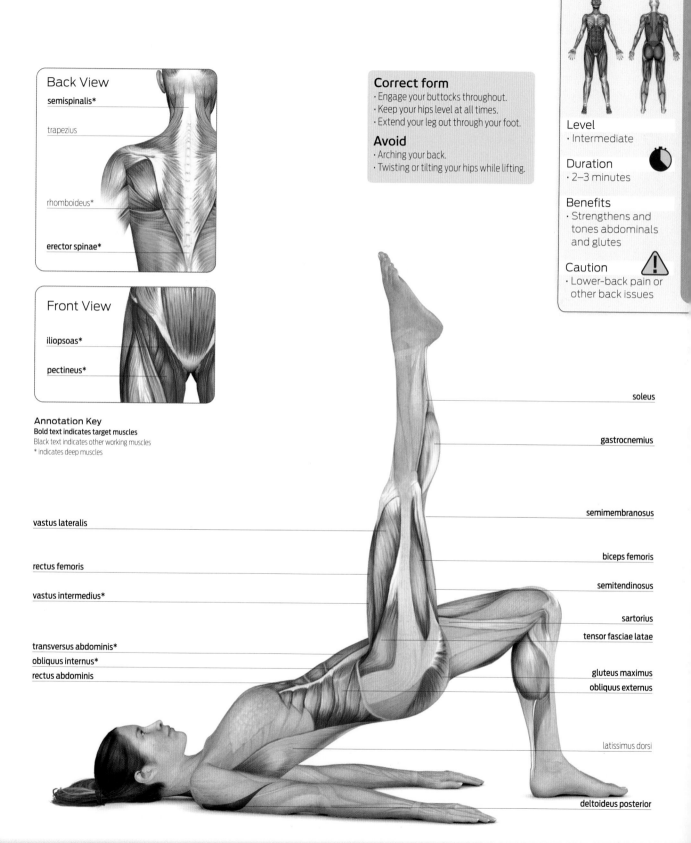

Back View

semispinalis*

trapezius

rhomboideus*

erector spinae*

Front View

iliopsoas*

pectineus*

Annotation Key
Bold text indicates target muscles
Black text indicates other working muscles
* indicates deep muscles

Correct form
- Engage your buttocks throughout.
- Keep your hips level at all times.
- Extend your leg out through your foot.

Avoid
- Arching your back.
- Twisting or tilting your hips while lifting.

Level
- Intermediate

Duration
- 2–3 minutes

Benefits
- Strengthens and tones abdominals and glutes

Caution
- Lower-back pain or other back issues

vastus lateralis

rectus femoris

vastus intermedius*

transversus abdominis*
obliquus internus*
rectus abdominis

soleus

gastrocnemius

semimembranosus

biceps femoris

semitendinosus

sartorius

tensor fasciae latae

gluteus maximus
obliquus externus

latissimus dorsi

deltoideus posterior

Side Leg Series

Getting the most out of Side Leg Series means keeping your core muscles completely still while your lower body moves: challenging, but well worth it. Over time you should achieve toned thighs and a sleeker, tighter midsection.

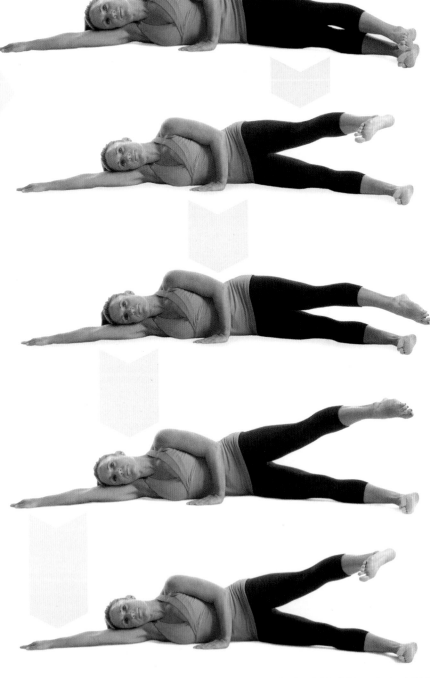

1 Lie on your side with your legs extended forward at a 45-degree angle to your body. Straighten your bottom arm and bend the other so that your hand is on the mat in front of you. Press your navel toward your spine and align your hips on top of each other.

2 Lift your top leg and flex your foot. From your hip joint, slightly rotate your foot toward the mat and move your leg up and down 25 times.

3 Next, point your foot and lift your leg, and then flex your foot and lower your leg. Complete 25 repetitions.

4 Next, lift your top leg no higher than your hip and flex your foot. Maintaining a strong flexed foot, perform 50 pulses.

5 Repeat the entire series up to 5 times on each side.

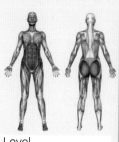

Front View

rectus abdominis

transversus abdominis*

iliopsoas*

pectineus*

sartorius

adductor brevis

adductor longus

gracilis*

vastus lateralis

vastus medialis

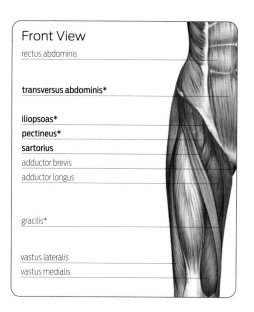

Back View

erector spinae*

quadratus lumborum*

gluteus minimus*

gluteus medius*

gluteus maximus

semitendinosus

biceps femoris

semimembranosus

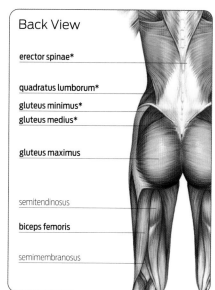

Level
· Intermediate

Duration

· 4–6 minutes

Benefits
· Strengthens and tightens core and quadriceps

Caution
· Hip issues

tensor fasciae latae

obliquus externus

rectus femoris

obliquus internus*

adductor longus

vastus intermedius*

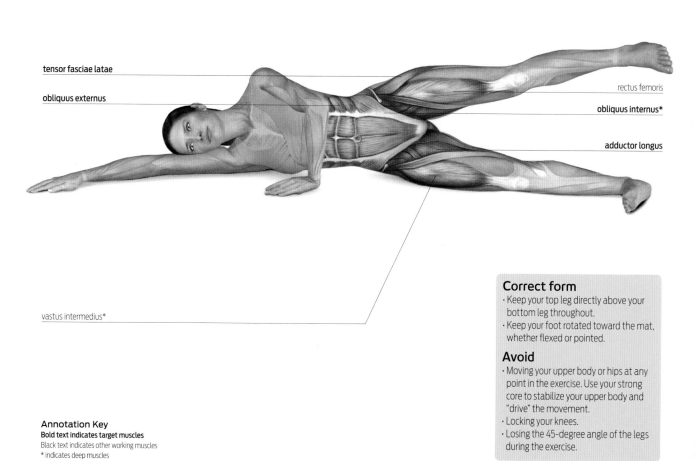

Correct form
· Keep your top leg directly above your bottom leg throughout.
· Keep your foot rotated toward the mat, whether flexed or pointed.

Avoid
· Moving your upper body or hips at any point in the exercise. Use your strong core to stabilize your upper body and "drive" the movement.
· Locking your knees.
· Losing the 45-degree angle of the legs during the exercise.

Annotation Key
Bold text indicates target muscles
Black text indicates other working muscles
* indicates deep muscles

Side-Lying Straight-Leg Circles

In Side-Lying Straight-Leg Circles, your legs are extended directly downward from your hips, rather than angled forward as in other side-lying exercises. The small leg circles strengthen and lengthen your legs, as well as improving your stability and honing your sense of balance.

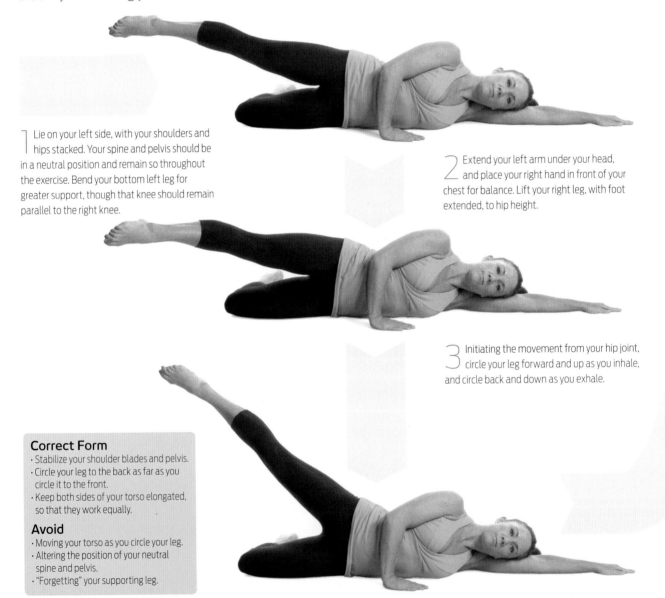

1 Lie on your left side, with your shoulders and hips stacked. Your spine and pelvis should be in a neutral position and remain so throughout the exercise. Bend your bottom left leg for greater support, though that knee should remain parallel to the right knee.

2 Extend your left arm under your head, and place your right hand in front of your chest for balance. Lift your right leg, with foot extended, to hip height.

3 Initiating the movement from your hip joint, circle your leg forward and up as you inhale, and circle back and down as you exhale.

Correct Form
· Stabilize your shoulder blades and pelvis.
· Circle your leg to the back as far as you circle it to the front.
· Keep both sides of your torso elongated, so that they work equally.

Avoid
· Moving your torso as you circle your leg.
· Altering the position of your neutral spine and pelvis.
· "Forgetting" your supporting leg.

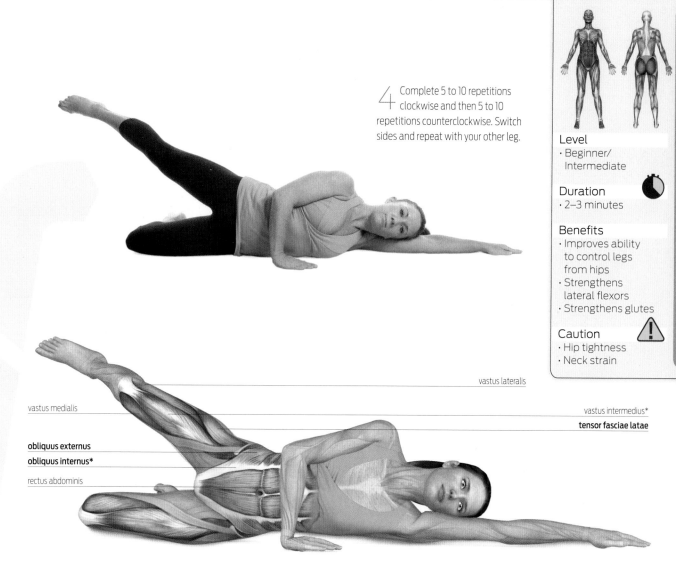

4 Complete 5 to 10 repetitions clockwise and then 5 to 10 repetitions counterclockwise. Switch sides and repeat with your other leg.

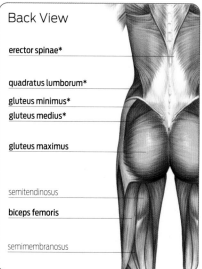

Level
· Beginner/ Intermediate

Duration
· 2–3 minutes

Benefits
· Improves ability to control legs from hips
· Strengthens lateral flexors
· Strengthens glutes

Caution
· Hip tightness
· Neck strain

vastus lateralis

vastus medialis

obliquus externus

obliquus internus*

rectus abdominis

vastus intermedius*

tensor fasciae latae

Annotation Key
Bold text indicates target muscles
Black text indicates other working muscles
* indicates deep muscles

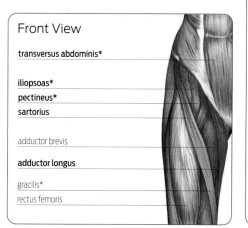

Front View

transversus abdominis*

iliopsoas*

pectineus*

sartorius

adductor brevis

adductor longus

gracilis*

rectus femoris

Back View

erector spinae*

quadratus lumborum*

gluteus minimus*

gluteus medius*

gluteus maximus

semitendinosus

biceps femoris

semimembranosus

Side-Lying Double-Leg Lift

This is yet another exercise in the side-lying series. As with the other exercises in this group, you'll work on moving your legs independently from your hips, which increases your range of motion and helps relieve pressure in your lower back while carrying out everyday movement.

Correct Form
· Stabilize your shoulder blades and pelvis.
· Pull up the front of your thighs.
· Keep both sides of your torso elongated, so they work equally.

Avoid
· Shifting shoulders and hips back and forth as you work your legs.
· Altering the position of your neutral spine and pelvis.

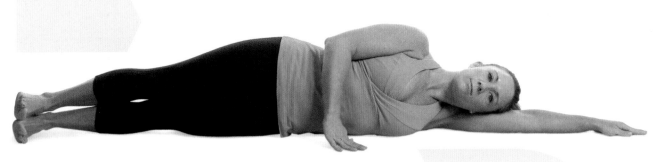

1 Lie on your left side, with your shoulders and hips stacked. Your spine and pelvis should be in a neutral position and remain so throughout the exercise.

2 Extend your left arm under your head, and place your right hand in front of your chest for balance. Flex your ankles and firmly press your inner thighs together. Inhale to prepare.

3 As you exhale, stretch your legs away from your upper body—so much so that your legs actually lift off the mat.

4 Inhale as you lower your legs to the mat again. Perform 5 to 10 repetitions, and then switch sides and repeat.

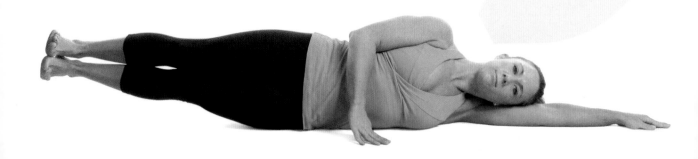

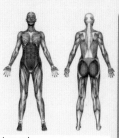

Modification

Harder: Perform the exercise with a ball pressed firmly between your feet, your ankles flexed. The ball adds resistance to your lower bodywork, increasing muscular engagement and awareness.

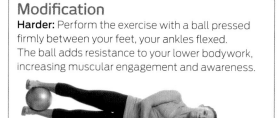

Back View

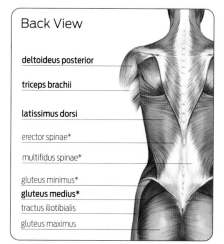

deltoideus posterior

triceps brachii

latissimus dorsi

erector spinae*

multifidus spinae*

gluteus minimus*

gluteus medius*

tractus iliotibialis

gluteus maximus

Level
· Beginner/ Intermediate

Duration
· 2–3 minutes

Benefits
· Improves ability to control legs from hips
· Strengthens lateral flexors
· Strengthens glutes

Caution
· Hip tightness
· Neck strain

Annotation Key
Bold text indicates target muscles
Black text indicates other working muscles
* indicates deep muscles

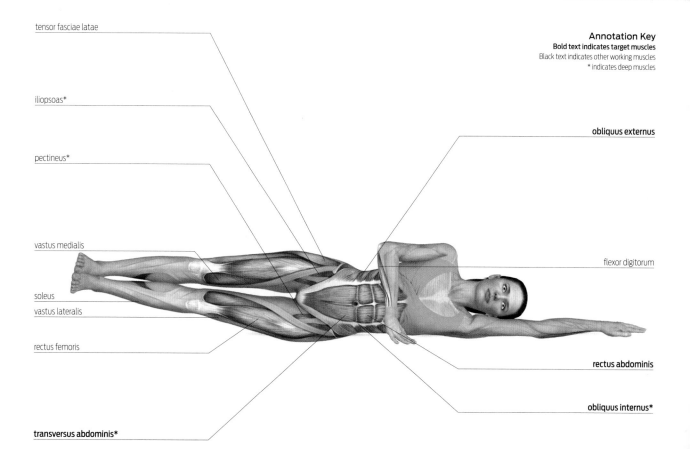

tensor fasciae latae

iliopsoas*

pectineus*

vastus medialis

soleus

vastus lateralis

rectus femoris

transversus abdominis*

obliquus externus

flexor digitorum

rectus abdominis

obliquus internus*

Pilates Ball Side-Lying Inner Thigh

Pilates Ball Side-Lying Inner Thigh strengthens and tones your hips, abdominals, and thighs. Keeping your hips and pelvis still as you pulse your leg is an exercise in core stability.

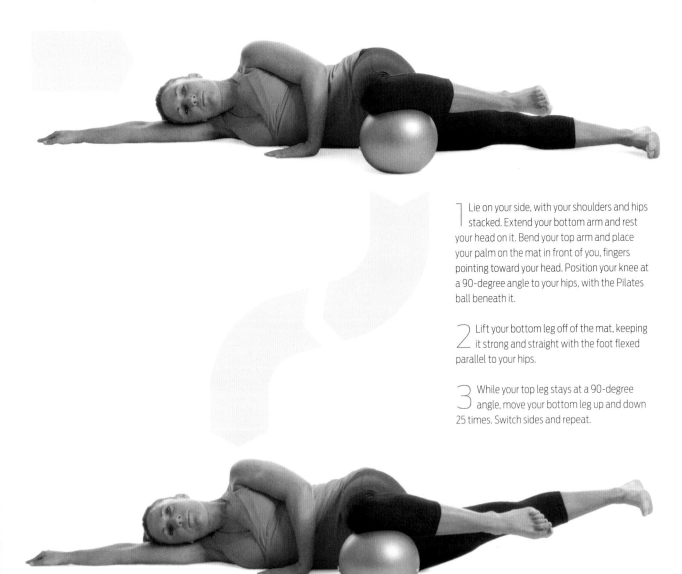

1 Lie on your side, with your shoulders and hips stacked. Extend your bottom arm and rest your head on it. Bend your top arm and place your palm on the mat in front of you, fingers pointing toward your head. Position your knee at a 90-degree angle to your hips, with the Pilates ball beneath it.

2 Lift your bottom leg off of the mat, keeping it strong and straight with the foot flexed parallel to your hips.

3 While your top leg stays at a 90-degree angle, move your bottom leg up and down 25 times. Switch sides and repeat.

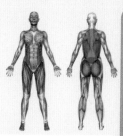

Back View

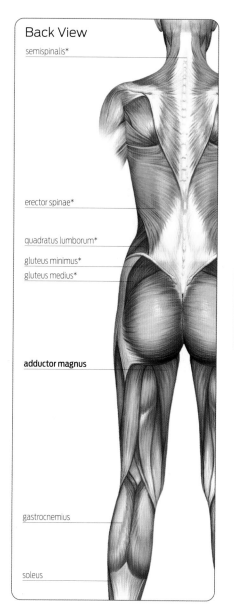

semispinalis*

erector spinae*

quadratus lumborum*

gluteus minimus*
gluteus medius*

adductor magnus

gastrocnemius

soleus

Correct form
· Engage your top leg to keep the ball in place.
· Keep your abdominal muscles and rib cage strongly compact.

Avoid
· Tensing your shoulders and/or neck.

Front View

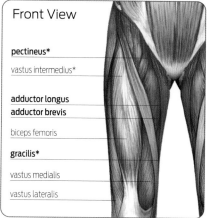

pectineus*

vastus intermedius*

adductor longus
adductor brevis

biceps femoris

gracilis*

vastus medialis

vastus lateralis

Level
· Intermediate

Duration
· 2–3 minutes

Benefits
· Strengthens and tones hips, abdominals, and thighs
· Stabilizes core

Caution
· Hip issues

Annotation Key
Bold text indicates target muscles
Black text indicates other working muscles
* indicates deep muscles

obliquus externus

obliquus internus*

Wide-Legged Plié

Borrowed from ballet training, Wide-Legged Plié targets your inner thighs and buttocks, helping you to attain lean and toned legs. It also strengthens your back muscles and abdominals and increases mobility in your hips.

3 Keeping your torso erect, slowly bend your knees, maintaining rotation in your legs.

1 Stand with your feet 2 to 3 feet apart, turned out from your hips. Your heels should be rotated forward, and your knees aligned directly over your feet.

2 Maintain a neutral pelvis as you press your navel toward your spine, using your abdominals to lift your arms out to the sides at shoulder height—and within your peripheral vision.

Correct form
· Keep your pelvis neutral and level.
· Press your shoulders down your back.
· Keep your weight slightly shifted toward your heels during the exercise to prevent your knees and feet from rolling in.

Avoid
· Allowing your knees to extend past your toes.
· Altering the position of your hips.
· Rotating your leg from the knees, instead of from the hips.
· Locking your knees.

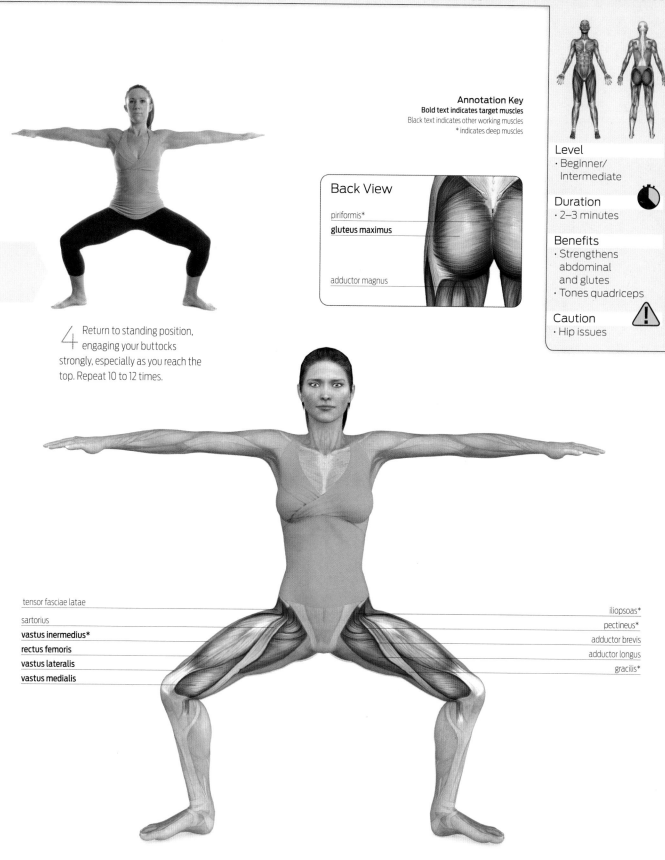

Annotation Key
Bold text indicates target muscles
Black text indicates other working muscles
* indicates deep muscles

Back View

piriformis*

gluteus maximus

adductor magnus

Level
· Beginner/
  Intermediate

Duration
· 2–3 minutes

Benefits
· Strengthens
  abdominal
  and glutes
· Tones quadriceps

Caution
· Hip issues

4 Return to standing position, engaging your buttocks strongly, especially as you reach the top. Repeat 10 to 12 times.

tensor fasciae latae
sartorius
vastus inermedius*
rectus femoris
vastus lateralis
vastus medialis

iliopsoas*
pectineus*
adductor brevis
adductor longus
gracilis*

Standing Leg Extension

Standing Leg Extension looks deceptively simple, but performing it correctly takes concentration. This exercise strengthens your quadriceps, that large group of muscles in the front of your thigh, and tones your abdominals and buttocks. It works your balance, too. While standing on one leg, it helps to focus your eyes on a spot in front of you.

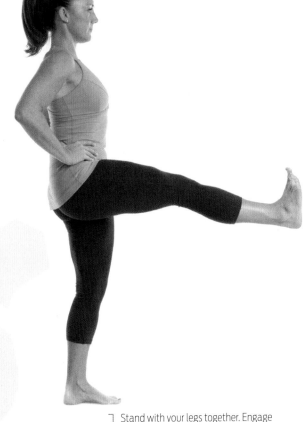

1 Stand with your legs together. Engage your abdominal muscles to stabilize your shoulders and your spine.

2 Glide your shoulders down your back to open your chest. Place your hands on your hips.

3 Bend one knee and lift your leg until your thigh is parallel to the mat, ankle flexed.

4 Keeping your ankle flexed, straighten your leg in front of you. Extend the leg only to a height at which you can continue to work the entire leg from the hip joint—while keeping your hips level.

5 Slowly bend your knee, returning it to a 90-degree angle. Complete 10 repetitions and then switch sides and repeat. Try to increase to 2 sets of 10 as you build up your strength and stamina.

Correct form
· Stabilize your torso.
· Engage your buttocks while extending your leg.
· Flex the ankle of your extended leg as if trying to see the sole of your shoe in the mirror.

Avoid
· Lifting your thigh higher than the level of your hip.
· Arching or collapsing your back.

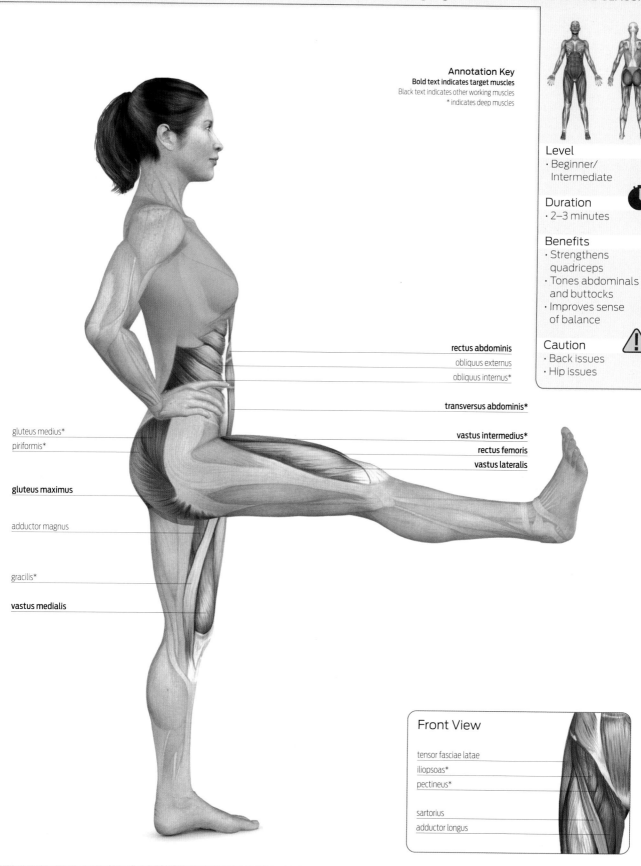

Annotation Key
Bold text indicates target muscles
Black text indicates other working muscles
* indicates deep muscles

Level
· Beginner/
  Intermediate

Duration
· 2–3 minutes

Benefits
· Strengthens
  quadriceps
· Tones abdominals
  and buttocks
· Improves sense
  of balance

Caution
· Back issues
· Hip issues

rectus abdominis
obliquus externus
obliquus internus*

transversus abdominis*

gluteus medius*
piriformis*

vastus intermedius*
rectus femoris
vastus lateralis

gluteus maximus

adductor magnus

gracilis*

vastus medialis

Front View

tensor fasciae latae
iliopsoas*
pectineus*

sartorius
adductor longus

Triceps Kick-Back

Triceps Kick-Back is an excellent, and relatively simple, exercise that tones your triceps. Keep your core strong and your whole body stable, even while you're balanced on two legs and just one arm.

1 Kneel on "all fours," with your wrists directly under your shoulders, your fingers facing forward, and your knees directly under your hips. (You can use a folded towel under your knees to relieve any discomfort.) Your spine and pelvis should be in neutral and your gaze toward the floor. Inhale as you press your navel toward your spine.

2 With your right hand in a fist—or holding a hand weight—exhale as you flex your elbow tightly into your side. Keep pressing your shoulder blades down your back.

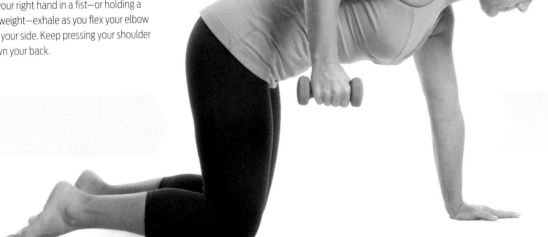

3 Inhale and slowly extend your right arm straight behind you, as if pulling on an elastic attached to the wall in front of you.

Correct Form
- Keep your pelvis and spine in a neutral position.
- Keep your line of sight toward the floor, so you don't shorten your cervical vertebrae.
- Hold your fist (or hand weight) directly under your shoulder.

Avoid
- Swinging your arm to move from one position to the next.
- Overextending your arm by locking your elbow.
- Relaxing your abdominals.

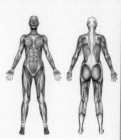

4 Exhale and slowly flex your elbow forward again, controlling the movement all the way. Repeat 10 times. Then, switch sides and repeat.

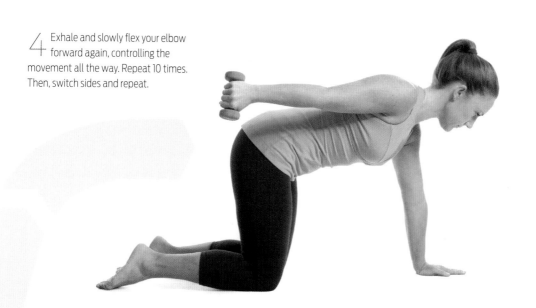

Level
· Beginner/ Intermediate

Duration
· 2–3 minutes

Benefits
· Strengthens triceps
· Develops control of upper body

Caution
· Elbow injury
· Lower-back issues

Annotation Key
Bold text indicates target muscles
Black text indicates other working muscles
* indicates deep muscles

deltoideus posterior

triceps brachii

rhomboideus*

serratus anterior

rectus abdominis

transversus abdominis*

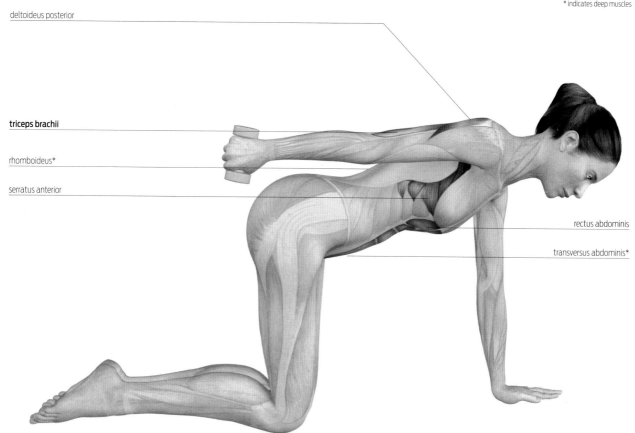

Triceps Push-Up

You've probably tried at least one of the plank-positioned exercises presented earlier in this book. Now it's time to use the plank position for a push-up. The push-up is a great exercise for all that might ail you: just see the list of muscles that are actively involved!

Correct Form
· Maintain your neutral spine and pelvis.
· Stabilize your shoulders down your back.
· Keep lifting up the front of your pelvis.
· Keep your legs strongly extended.

Avoid
· Lifting your pelvis, or allowing it to sink.
· Letting your belly sink toward the mat.
· Placing your elbows too close to your body.

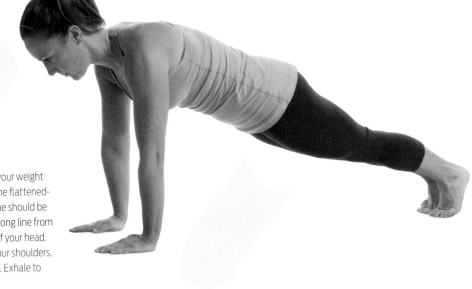

1 Assume a plank position with your weight on the balls on your feet and the flattened-out palms of your hands. Your spine should be in a neutral position, forming one long line from your tailbone through the crown of your head. Your wrists are directly beneath your shoulders, with your fingers pointing forward. Exhale to prepare.

2 Inhale as you slowly bend your elbows, lowering your torso toward the mat.

3 Exhale as you extend your elbows to raise your plank-positioned body up again. Complete 4 to 10 repetitions.

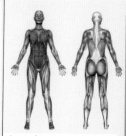

Modification

Easier: Start on your hands and knees, with your wrists aligned beneath your shoulder. Lift your feet toward your buttocks until your calves and thighs form a 90-degree angle.

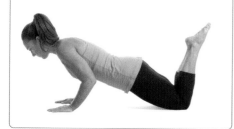

Annotation Key
Bold text indicates target muscles
Black text indicates other working muscles
* indicates deep muscles

erector spinae*

deltoideus posterior

trapezius

biceps brachii

Front View

deltoideus anterior

pectoralis minor

coracobrachialis*

pectoralis major

serratus anterior

obliquus internus*

rectus abdominis

transversus abdominis*

vastus intermedius*

rectus femoris

vastus lateralis

vastus medialis

Level
· Intermediate

Duration
· 2–4 minutes

Benefits
· Stabilizes core muscles
· Strengthens abdominals
· Enhances awareness of full body integration

Caution
· Lower-back pain
· Shoulder issues
· Wrist weakness

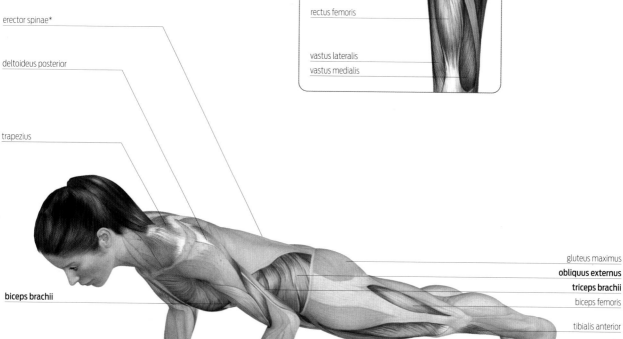

gluteus maximus

obliquus externus

triceps brachii

biceps femoris

tibialis anterior

Triceps Dip

You'll really feel the effects of Triceps Dip on the backs of your arms when you do this exercise correctly. This dip engages everything else, too, due to the effort that's needed to keep your body in position. Balancing on your heels throughout the exercise pushes your body weight toward your upper body so that your triceps have to work harder to support you.

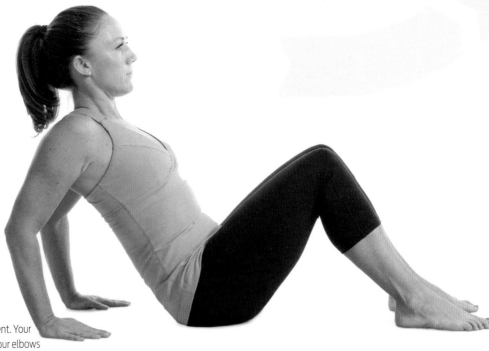

1 Sit on your mat with your knees bent. Your arms should be behind you with your elbows bent and the palms of your hands pressing into the mat, fingers facing forward. Straighten your arms as you lift your hips a few inches off the mat.

2 Shift your weight back toward your arms, and, keeping your heels pressed firmly into the mat, lift your toes.

3 Bend your elbows, keeping your chest open and your gaze diagonally upward.

Correct form
· Keep your chest lifted and open.
· Hold your shoulders down.

Avoid
· Arching your back.
· Lifting your shoulders.
· Rushing through the exercise.

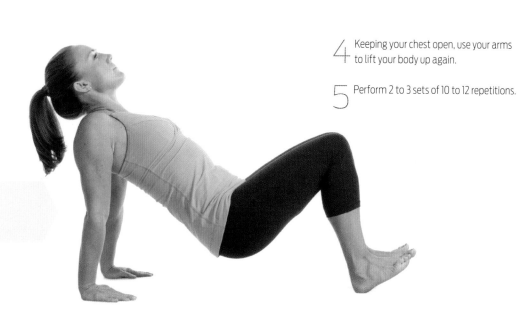

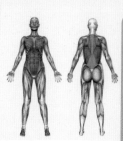

4 Keeping your chest open, use your arms to lift your body up again.

5 Perform 2 to 3 sets of 10 to 12 repetitions.

Level
· Advanced

Duration
· 2–3 minutes

Benefits
· Strengthens triceps, shoulders, chest, back, and core
· Tones abs

Caution
· Back issues
· Shoulder issues

Annotation Key
Bold text indicates target muscles
Black text indicates other working muscles
* indicates deep muscles

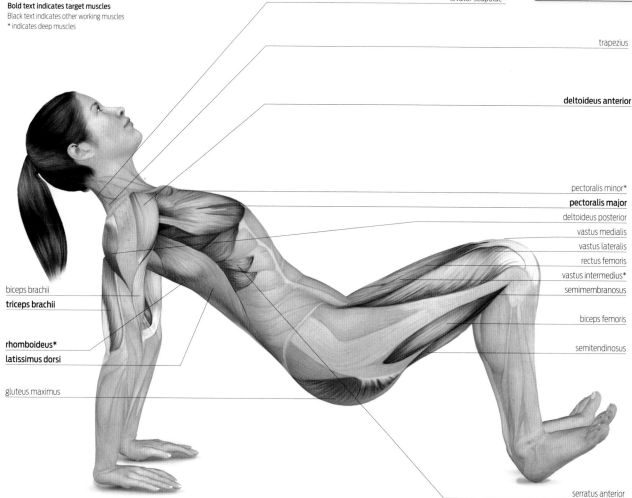

levator scapulae*

trapezius

deltoideus anterior

pectoralis minor*

pectoralis major

deltoideus posterior

vastus medialis

vastus lateralis

rectus femoris

vastus intermedius*

semimembranosus

biceps femoris

semitendinosus

serratus anterior

biceps brachii

triceps brachii

rhomboideus*

latissimus dorsi

gluteus maximus

Chest Fly

Chest Fly is a fairly simple though quite effective
exercise that works your major chest muscles.
Since physical movement is isolated in your arms,
this exercise offers the opportunity to focus on
scapulae and pelvis stabilization. Hand weights are used.

1 Lie on your back with your spine and pelvis
in a neutral position. Your knees should
be bent, parallel, and hip-distant from each
other. Extend your arms out to your sides, level
with your shoulders. Make sure your elbows
aren't locked. Hold the weights in your hands,
palms facing the ceiling. Exhale and press your
navel back toward your spine.

2 Inhale as you lift your arms in a c-curve
until the weights touch each other in
front of your chest.

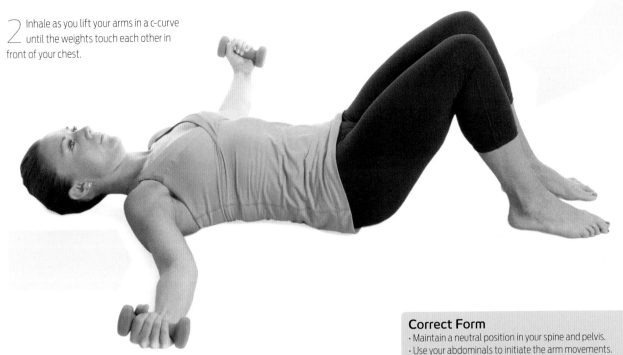

Correct Form
· Maintain a neutral position in your spine and pelvis.
· Use your abdominals to initiate the arm movements.
· Maintain a compact, strong rib cage.

Avoid
· Arching your neck.
· Popping your arms forward from your shoulder sockets.
· Letting your arms completely relax on the floor when
  you open your arms.
· Locking your elbows.

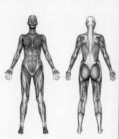

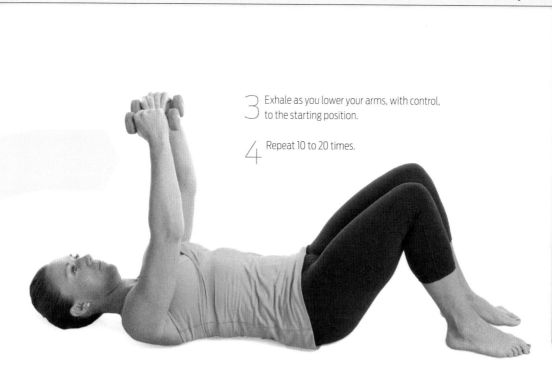

3 Exhale as you lower your arms, with control, to the starting position.

4 Repeat 10 to 20 times.

Level
· Beginner

Duration
· 2–3 minutes

Benefits
· Strengthens upper back, shoulders, and upper arms
· Stretches chest muscles

Caution
· Elbow injury

Back View

deltoideus posterior

subscapularis*

Annotation Key
Bold text indicates target muscles
Black text indicates other working muscles
* indicates deep muscles

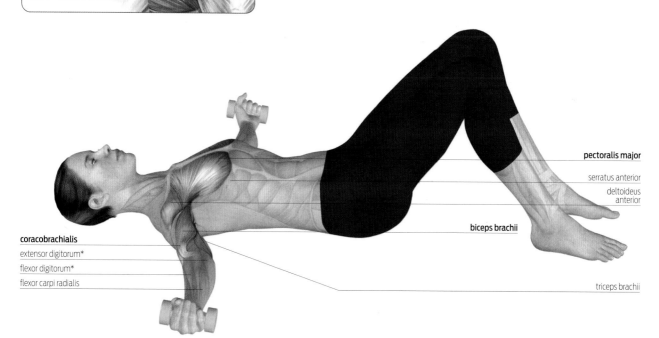

pectoralis major

serratus anterior

deltoideus anterior

biceps brachii

coracobrachialis

extensor digitorum*

flexor digitorum*

flexor carpi radialis

triceps brachii

Back Extension

Back Extension works your triceps and biceps, opens your chest, and firmly plugs your shoulder blades down your back. Hand weights are used. You might want to do this exercise standing on the floor, where your feet have a firm grip.

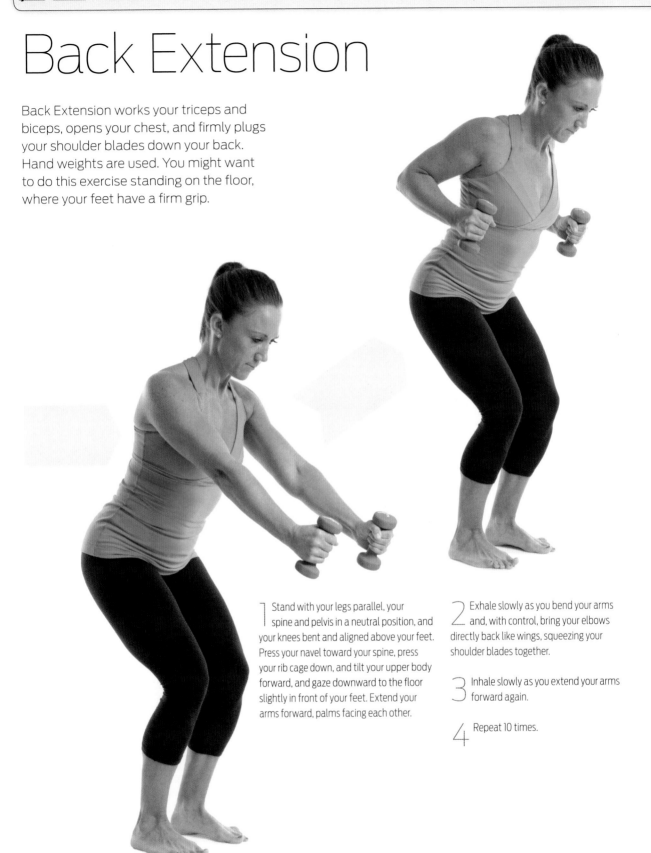

1 Stand with your legs parallel, your spine and pelvis in a neutral position, and your knees bent and aligned above your feet. Press your navel toward your spine, press your rib cage down, and tilt your upper body forward, and gaze downward to the floor slightly in front of your feet. Extend your arms forward, palms facing each other.

2 Exhale slowly as you bend your arms and, with control, bring your elbows directly back like wings, squeezing your shoulder blades together.

3 Inhale slowly as you extend your arms forward again.

4 Repeat 10 times.

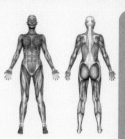

Correct Form
· Keep your chest open.
· Stabilize your shoulder blades.
· Keep your legs parallel.

Avoid
· Overarching your lumbar spine.
· Allowing your rib cage to pop outward.

Annotation Key
Bold text indicates target muscles
Black text indicates other working muscles
* indicates deep muscles

Level
· Beginner

Duration
· 2–3 minutes

Benefits
· Strengthens and stretches triceps
· Promotes awareness of scapulae

Caution
· Elbow injury
· Lower-back issues

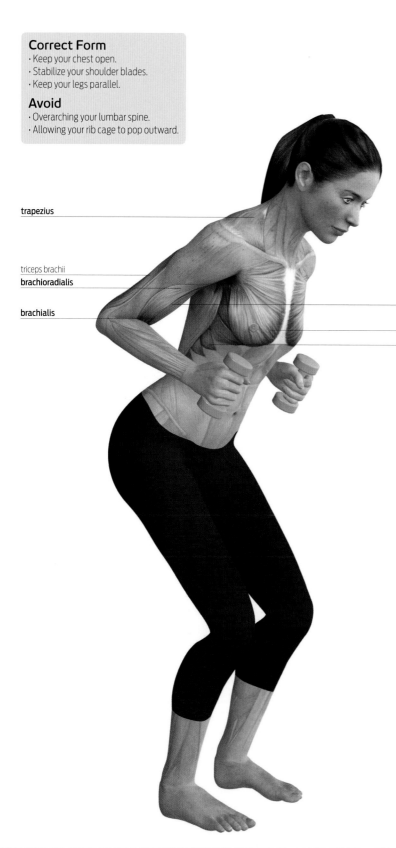

trapezius

triceps brachii
brachioradialis

brachialis

biceps brachii

pectoralis major
serratus anterior

Back View

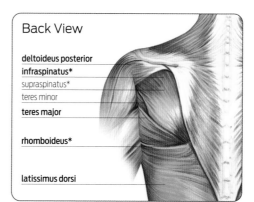

deltoideus posterior
infraspinatus*
supraspinatus*
teres minor
teres major

rhomboideus*

latissimus dorsi

Reverse Hug

Also called Reverse Fly, Reverse Hug uses hand weights and works your upper back, shoulders, and arms. Stand on the floor, rather than your mat, for greater stability.

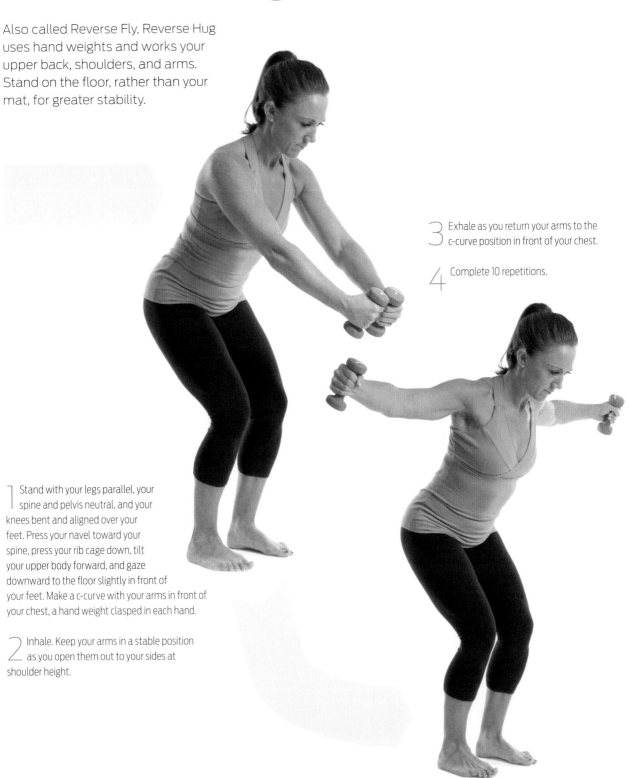

3 Exhale as you return your arms to the c-curve position in front of your chest.

4 Complete 10 repetitions.

1 Stand with your legs parallel, your spine and pelvis neutral, and your knees bent and aligned over your feet. Press your navel toward your spine, press your rib cage down, tilt your upper body forward, and gaze downward to the floor slightly in front of your feet. Make a c-curve with your arms in front of your chest, a hand weight clasped in each hand.

2 Inhale. Keep your arms in a stable position as you open them out to your sides at shoulder height.

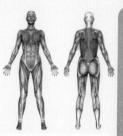

Correct Form
· Lift your elbows equally high as you open them outward.
· Stabilize your arms from under your shoulder blades as you curve inward.

Avoid
· Moving your upper body as you move your arms.
· Altering the position of your wrists.

Annotation Key
Bold text indicates target muscles
Black text indicates other working muscles
* indicates deep muscles

Level
· Beginner

Duration
· 2–3 minutes

Benefits
· Strengthens upper back and shoulders
· Stretches chest muscles

Caution
· Neck issues
· Shoulder injury

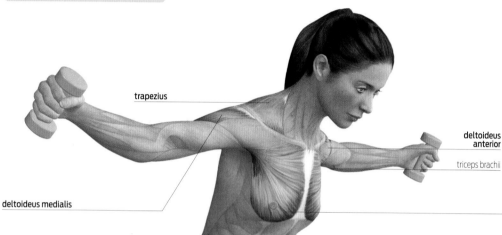

trapezius

deltoideus anterior

triceps brachii

deltoideus medialis

pectoralis major

Back View

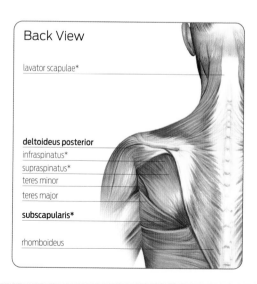

lavator scapulae*

deltoideus posterior
infraspinatus*
supraspinatus*
teres minor
teres major
subscapularis*
rhomboideus

Shoulder Press

Shoulder Press works your upper body, especially the deltoids and triceps. Sense the total body integration of movement as you work your arms, and notice the extra challenges that are presented when you exercise standing up.

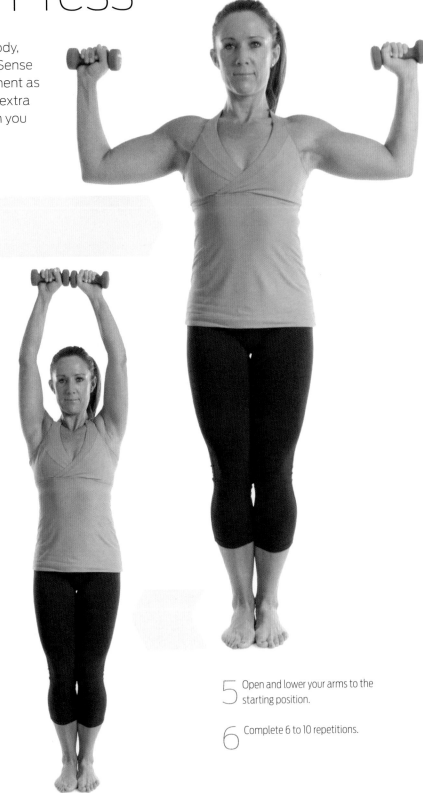

1 Stand with your legs together, spine and pelvis in a neutral position.

2 With your weights in your hands, extend your arms directly out to your sides at shoulder level.

3 Bend your elbows so that your arms form roughly 90-degree angles, with palms facing forward.

4 Keeping your shoulder blades pressed firmly down your back, raise your arms overhead so that the weights meet.

5 Open and lower your arms to the starting position.

6 Complete 6 to 10 repetitions.

Correct Form
· Maintain your neutral pelvis and spine position.
· Press your shoulder blades down your back.
· Work your arms from underneath your back.

Avoid
· Tensing your neck muscles
· Jutting your chin forward.
· Allowing your elbows to sink below shoulder height.

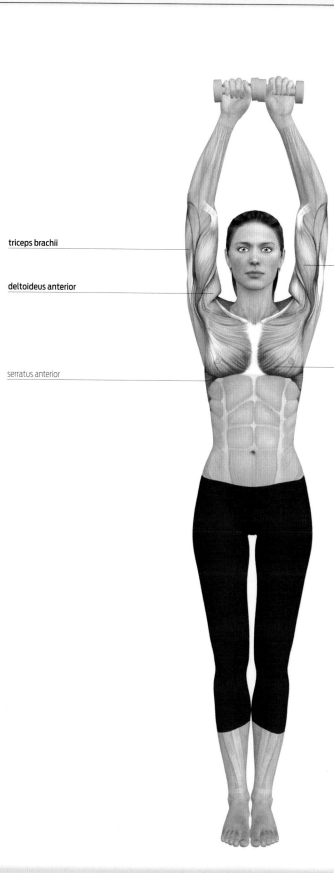

Annotation Key
Bold text indicates target muscles
Black text indicates other working muscles
* indicates deep muscles

triceps brachii

deltoideus anterior

serratus anterior

biceps brachii

pectoralis major

Level
· Beginner

Duration
· 2–3 minutes

Benefits
· Strengthens arms
· Develops shoulder muscles
· Opens and stretches chest

Caution
· Elbow issues
· Shoulder injury

Back View

lavator scapulae*

deltoideus posterior
infraspinatus*
supraspinatus*
teres minor
teres major
subscapularis*

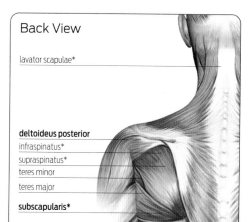

Shoulder Raise

Shoulder Raise works your upper body—the chest, shoulders, shoulder blades, and upper back. Remember that muscles move in opposition, which means that movement in one direction is accompanied by an equally strong movement in the opposite direction. Visualize lifting your shoulders by pressing your shoulder blades down your back.

1 Stand with your legs together, with your spine and pelvis in a neutral position.

2 Holding small hand weights, extend your arms directly out to your sides at shoulder level, palms facing the floor. Inhale to press your navel toward your spine.

3 Exhale while lifting your shoulder girdle slightly upward.

Correct Form
· Maintain your neutral pelvis and spine position.
· Keep your chest open.
· Engage your abdominals throughout the exercise.

Avoid
· Rolling your shoulders forward.
· Jutting your chin forward.
· Relaxing your wrists.

Modification
Harder: To challenge your core stability, balance, and coordination, stand on your right leg with your ankle strongly flexed. Lower your left arm, lift it to your side, and then repeat with your right arm. Perform 2 to 4 sets. Switch your standing leg and repeat.

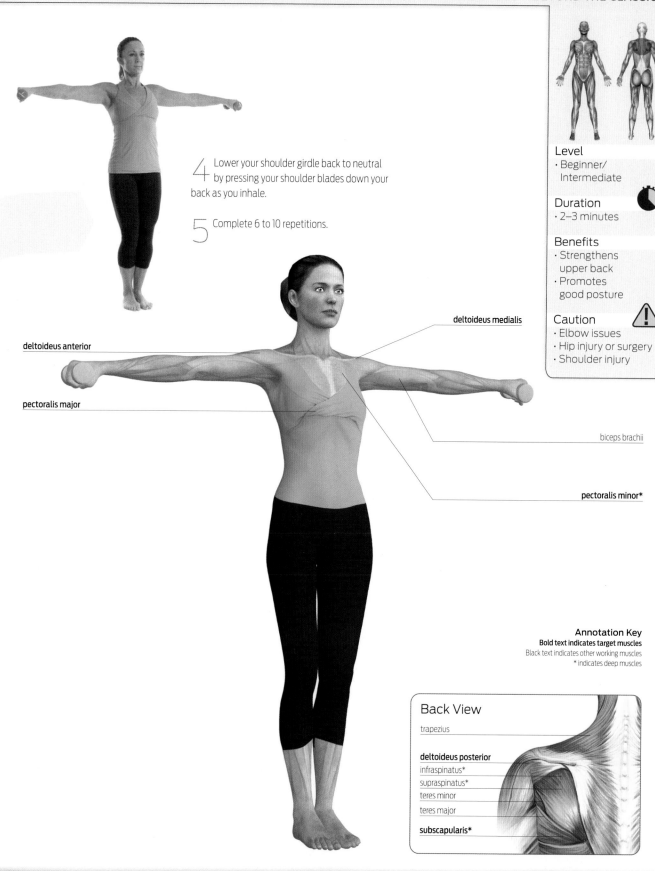

4 Lower your shoulder girdle back to neutral by pressing your shoulder blades down your back as you inhale.

5 Complete 6 to 10 repetitions.

deltoideus medialis

deltoideus anterior

pectoralis major

biceps brachii

pectoralis minor*

Level
· Beginner/ Intermediate

Duration
· 2–3 minutes

Benefits
· Strengthens upper back
· Promotes good posture

Caution
· Elbow issues
· Hip injury or surgery
· Shoulder injury

Annotation Key
Bold text indicates target muscles
Black text indicates other working muscles
* indicates deep muscles

Back View

trapezius

deltoideus posterior
infraspinatus*
supraspinatus*
teres minor
teres major
subscapularis*

Ballet Biceps

Ballet Biceps is a variation on the Shoulder Press exercise. This time, you're working with rounded arms that curve through the space, instead of angular arms that press up through the space. Your upward position should resemble the fifth position in ballet, with your arms extended above your head.

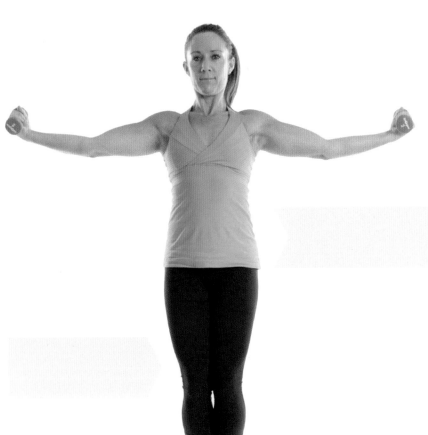

1 Stand with your legs together, spine and pelvis in a neutral position.

2 With your weights in your hands, extend your arms directly out to your sides at shoulder level. Relax your elbows slightly so your arms form gentle, though strong, curves.

3 Inhale as you lift your arms out to your sides and up overhead to frame your neck and head.

4 Exhale as you open and lower your arms to the start position.

5 Complete 6 to 10 repetitions.

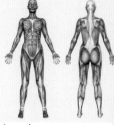

Correct Form
· Maintain your neutral pelvis and spine position.
· Stabilize your shoulders down your back.
· Keep the shape of your arms strongly held.

Avoid
· Tensing your neck muscles.
· Lifting your shoulders.
· Rolling your shoulders forward.

Annotation Key
Bold text indicates target muscles
Black text indicates other working muscles
* indicates deep muscles

Level
· Beginner

Duration
· 2–3 minutes

Benefits
· Strengthens and stretches arms
· Develops shoulder muscles
· Softens pressure on joints while increasing upper-body strength

Caution
· Elbow issues
· Shoulder injury

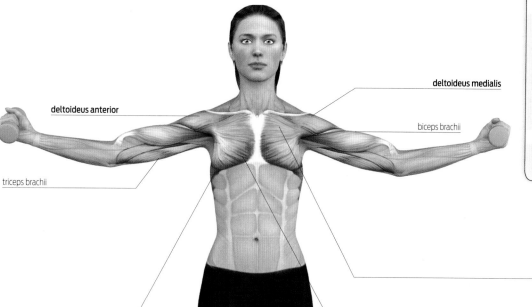

deltoideus anterior

deltoideus medialis

biceps brachii

triceps brachii

serratus anterior

pectoralis minor*

pectoralis major

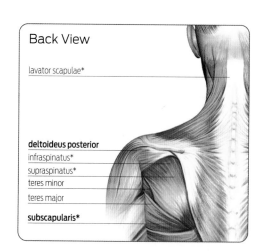

Back View

lavator scapulae*

deltoideus posterior
infraspinatus*
supraspinatus*
teres minor
teres major
subscapularis*

The Zipper

The Zipper develops your upper-body strength while reinforcing its connection to lower-body stability. In this exercise, you move as if you were unzipping a jacket and then pulling it wide open.

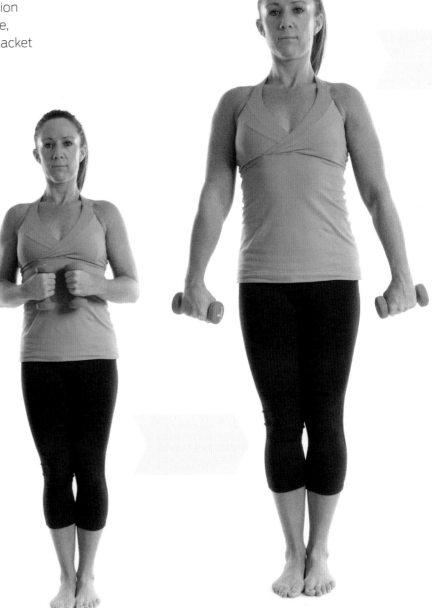

1 Stand with your legs together, spine and pelvis in a neutral position.

2 Holding your hand weights, bend your elbows and place your hands together right below your bottom ribs. Keep your elbows close to your sides.

3 "Zip" down the midline of your body with the fists of your hands together.

Correct Form
· Maintain your neutral posture.
· Press your shoulders down your back.
· Make the zipping movement strong.
· Keep your chest open.

Avoid
· Letting your shoulders roll forward.
· Breaking your rhythm or losing momentum.
· "Forgetting" your lower body.

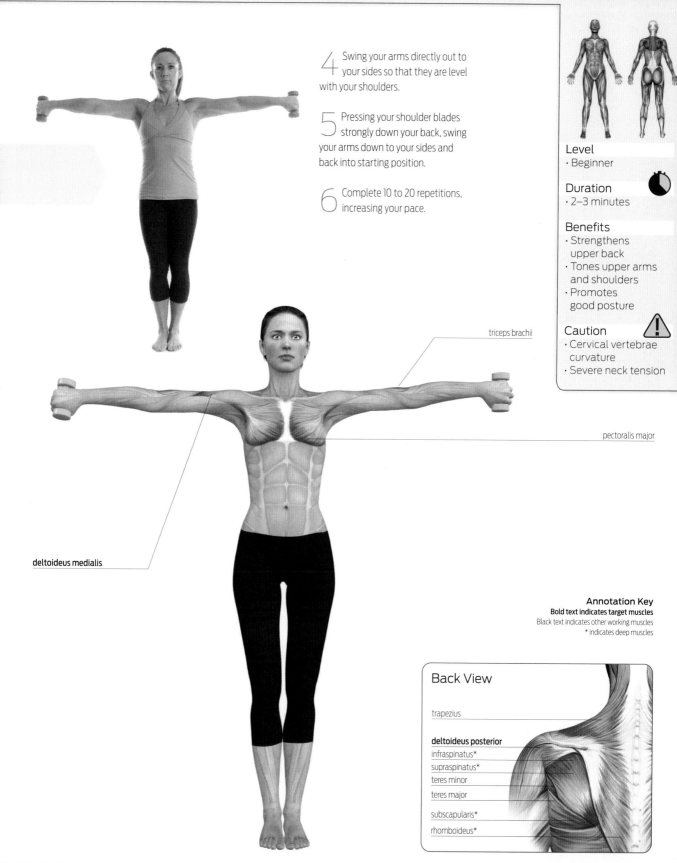

4 Swing your arms directly out to your sides so that they are level with your shoulders.

5 Pressing your shoulder blades strongly down your back, swing your arms down to your sides and back into starting position.

6 Complete 10 to 20 repetitions, increasing your pace.

Level
· Beginner

Duration
· 2–3 minutes

Benefits
· Strengthens upper back
· Tones upper arms and shoulders
· Promotes good posture

Caution
· Cervical vertebrae curvature
· Severe neck tension

triceps brachii

pectoralis major

deltoideus medialis

Annotation Key
Bold text indicates target muscles
Black text indicates other working muscles
* indicates deep muscles

Back View

trapezius

deltoideus posterior
infraspinatus*
supraspinatus*
teres minor
teres major
subscapularis*
rhomboideus*

Basic Biceps Curl

Basic Biceps Curl is simple. Take your time while working on it, picturing your joints attached to the walls of your workout space by long, strong elastics. Think of resistance as well as fluidity as you move.

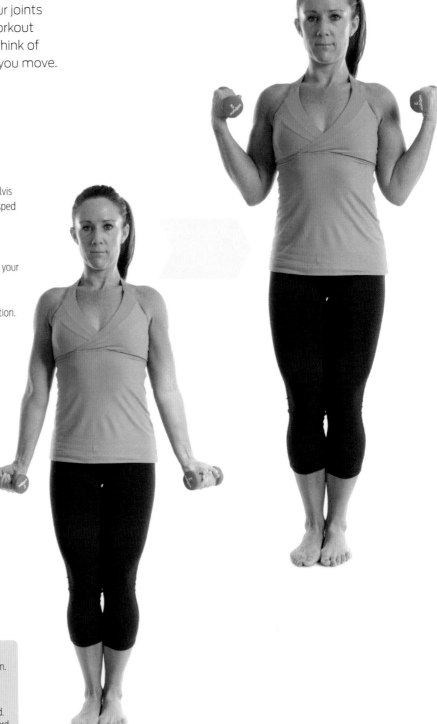

1 Stand with your legs together, spine and pelvis in a neutral position. With your weights clasped in your hands, extend your arms down by your sides.

2 Inhale as you bend your elbows and press your lower arms upward your shoulders.

3 Exhale as you return to your starting position.

4 Complete 6 to 10 repetitions.

Correct Form
· Maintain your neutral pelvis and spine position.
· Keep your elbows close to your sides.

Avoid
· Lifting your shoulders, or rolling them forward.
· Twisting your wrists either forward or backward.

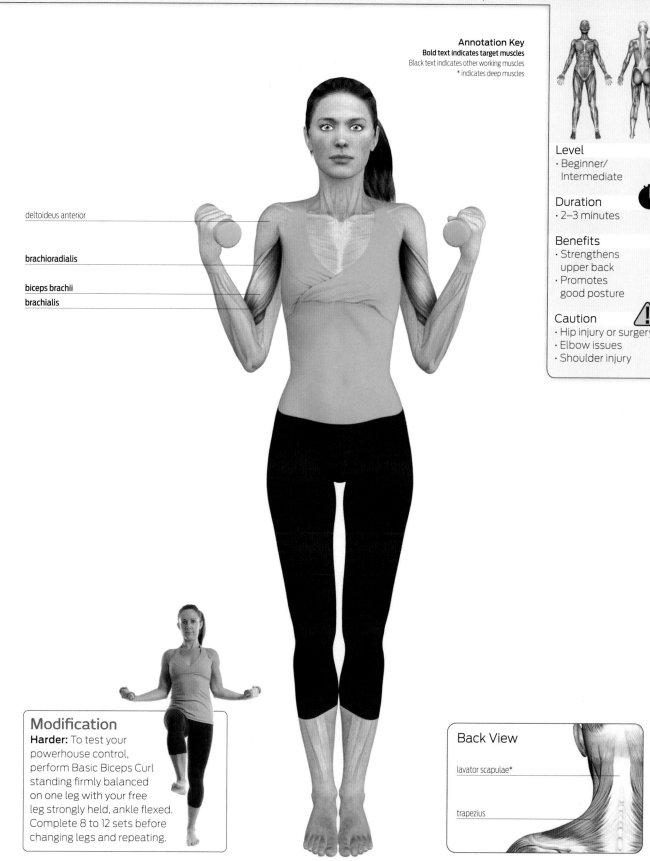

Annotation Key
Bold text indicates target muscles
Black text indicates other working muscles
* indicates deep muscles

deltoideus anterior

brachioradialis

biceps brachii
brachialis

Level
· Beginner/
  Intermediate

Duration
· 2–3 minutes

Benefits
· Strengthens
  upper back
· Promotes
  good posture

Caution
· Hip injury or surgery
· Elbow issues
· Shoulder injury

Modification

Harder: To test your powerhouse control, perform Basic Biceps Curl standing firmly balanced on one leg with your free leg strongly held, ankle flexed. Complete 8 to 12 sets before changing legs and repeating.

Back View

lavator scapulae*

trapezius

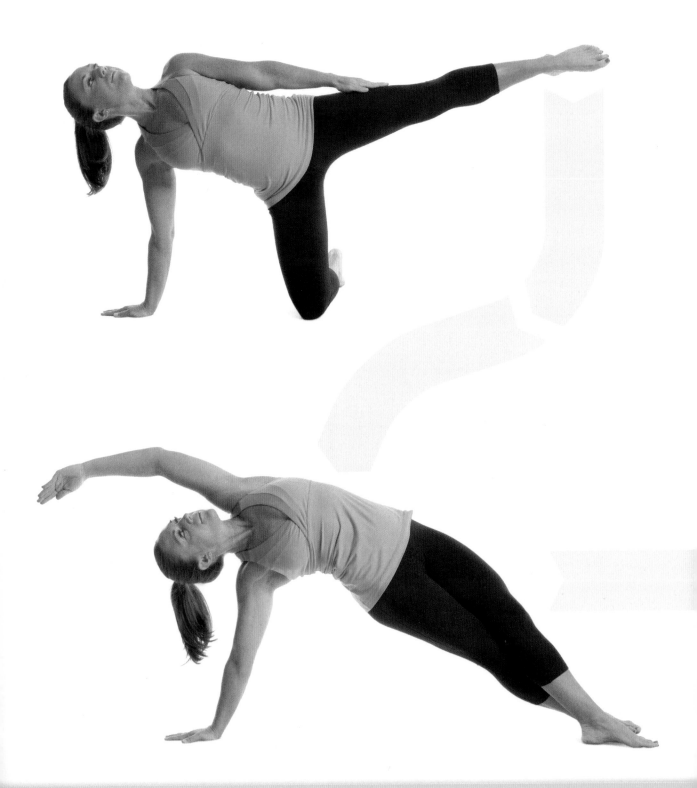

Workouts

One of the satisfying aspects of Pilates practice is that it targets your whole body. When performed with correct form and some regularity, the following sequences not only work body parts like backs, arms, and core, but they also make your entire physique sleeker and stronger along the way. Try mixing and matching among the different sequences until you find a routine that challenges you. Don't forget to keep breathing throughout your workout.

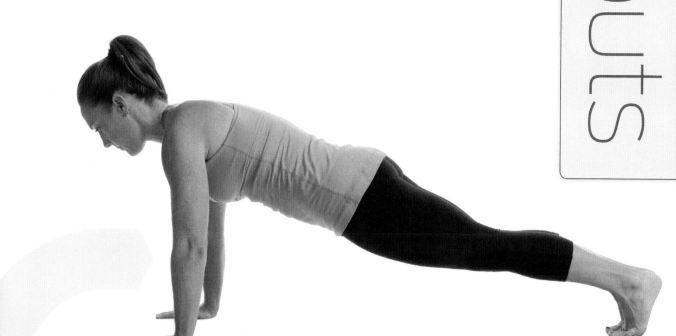

Contents

Classical Pilates I

This series of exercises gives you a sense of the progression of a traditional Pilates routine. It's an excellent way to work your abdominal muscles and move your spine.

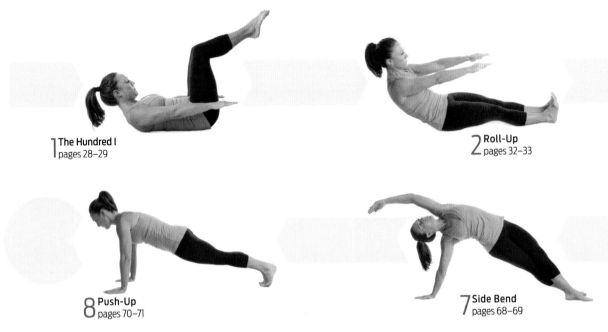

1 **The Hundred I**
pages 28–29

2 **Roll-Up**
pages 32–33

8 **Push-Up**
pages 70–71

7 **Side Bend**
pages 68–69

Classical Pilates II

This series offers another sequence of traditional Pilates exercises. If you let one exercise flow into the next and pick up the pace, you'll find yourself both warm and invigorated when you're finished.

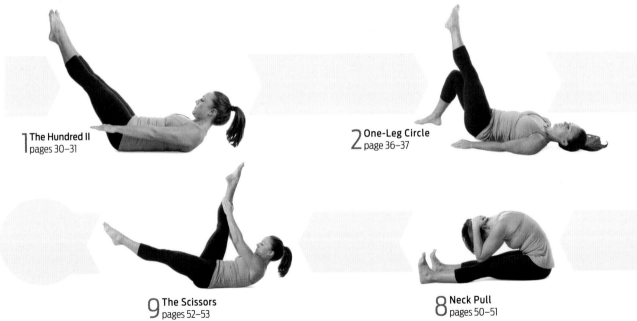

1 **The Hundred II**
pages 30–31

2 **One-Leg Circle**
page 36–37

9 **The Scissors**
pages 52–53

8 **Neck Pull**
pages 50–51

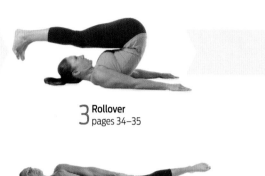

3 **Rollover**
pages 34–35

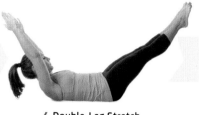

4 **Double-Leg Stretch**
pages 42–43

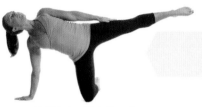

6 **Side Leg Kick Kneeling**
pages 66–67

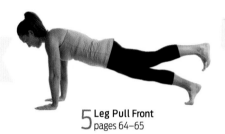

5 **Leg Pull Front**
pages 64–65

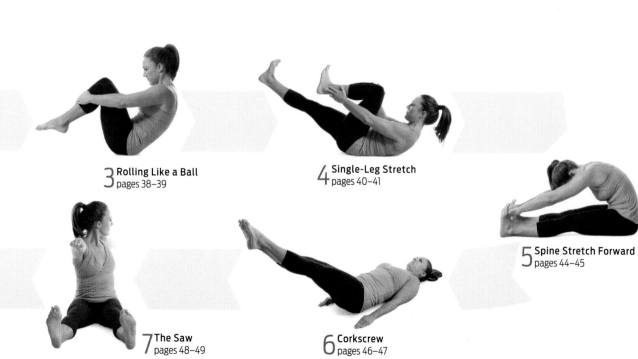

3 **Rolling Like a Ball**
pages 38–39

4 **Single-Leg Stretch**
pages 40–41

5 **Spine Stretch Forward**
pages 44–45

7 **The Saw**
pages 48–49

6 **Corkscrew**
pages 46–47

Advanced Core I

You can't beat Pilates for rigorously working your powerhouse. If you carry out the following workouts on a regular basis, a sleeker, tighter, stronger midsection will be your reward.

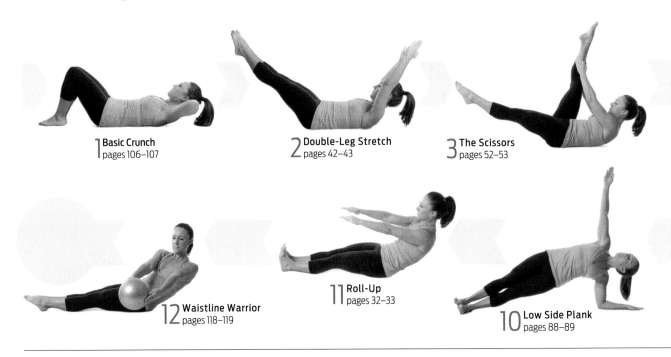

1 **Basic Crunch**
pages 106–107

2 **Double-Leg Stretch**
pages 42–43

3 **The Scissors**
pages 52–53

12 **Waistline Warrior**
pages 118–119

11 **Roll-Up**
pages 32–33

10 **Low Side Plank**
pages 88–89

Advanced Core II

If you follow Advanced Core I followed by Advanced Core II in a single session, you should definitely feel results. Otherwise, alternate between the two workouts throughout the week to add variety to your core regimen.

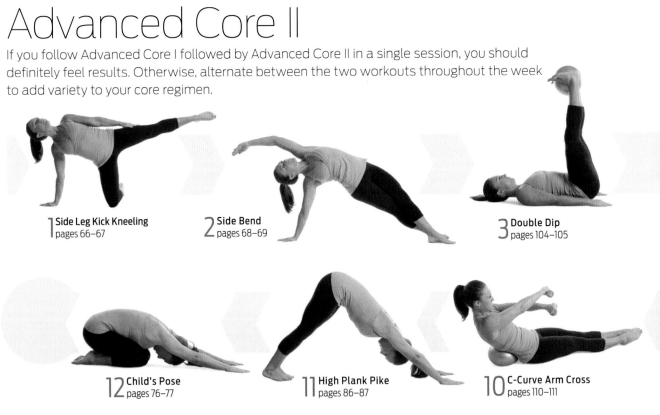

1 **Side Leg Kick Kneeling**
pages 66–67

2 **Side Bend**
pages 68–69

3 **Double Dip**
pages 104–105

12 **Child's Pose**
pages 76–77

11 **High Plank Pike**
pages 86–87

10 **C-Curve Arm Cross**
pages 110–111

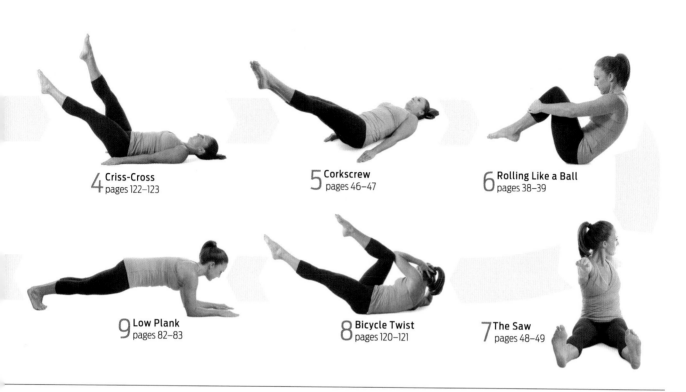

4 Criss-Cross
pages 122–123

5 Corkscrew
pages 46–47

6 Rolling Like a Ball
pages 38–39

9 Low Plank
pages 82–83

8 Bicycle Twist
pages 120–121

7 The Saw
pages 48–49

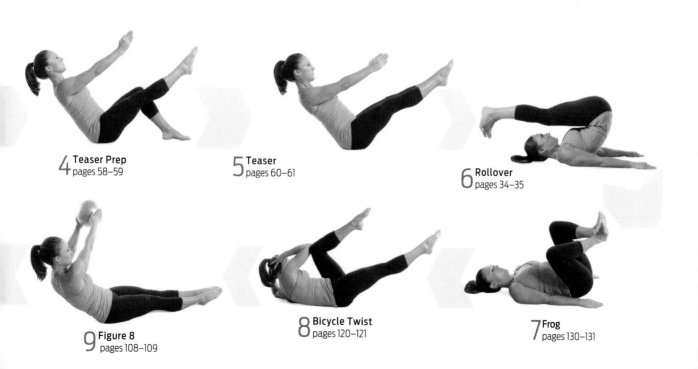

4 Teaser Prep
pages 58–59

5 Teaser
pages 60–61

6 Rollover
pages 34–35

9 Figure 8
pages 108–109

8 Bicycle Twist
pages 120–121

7 Frog
pages 130–131

Side-Lying Workout

All of the exercise in the sequence start in the side-lying position and demand a still core. The payout for proper form will be toned legs and trim midsection.

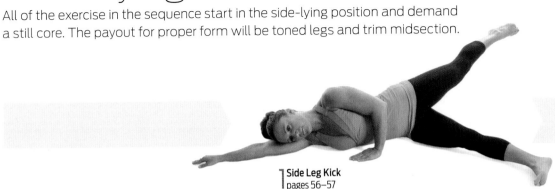

1 **Side Leg Kick**
pages 56–57

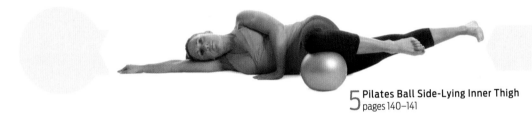

5 **Pilates Ball Side-Lying Inner Thigh**
pages 140–141

Working the Leg–Core Connection

This sequence, done lying on your back or your side, automatically offers your core the support of the floor so that you can work your legs from deep in your hip socks. The more you use your powerhouse muscles, the greater the ease of movement and power in your legs.

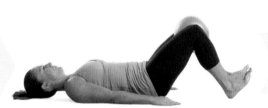

1 **Pilates Ball Heel Taps** pages 126–127

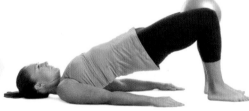

2 **Pilates Ball Tabletop-Bridge** pages 112–113

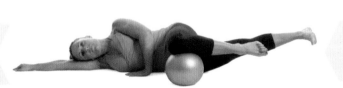

7 **Pilates Ball Side-Lying Inner Thigh**
pages 140–141

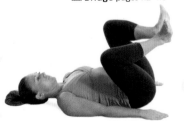

6 **Frog**
pages 130–131

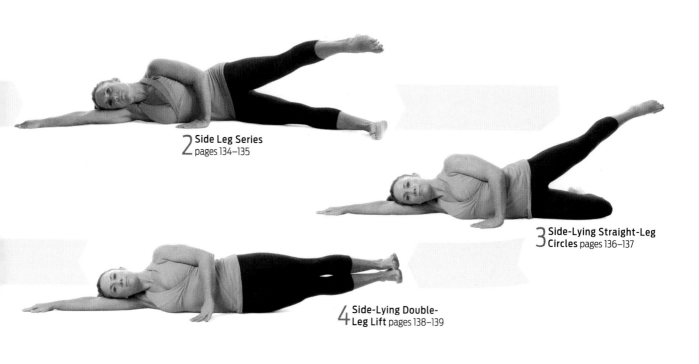

2 **Side Leg Series**
pages 134–135

3 **Side-Lying Straight-Leg**
Circles pages 136–137

4 **Side-Lying Double-**
Leg Lift pages 138–139

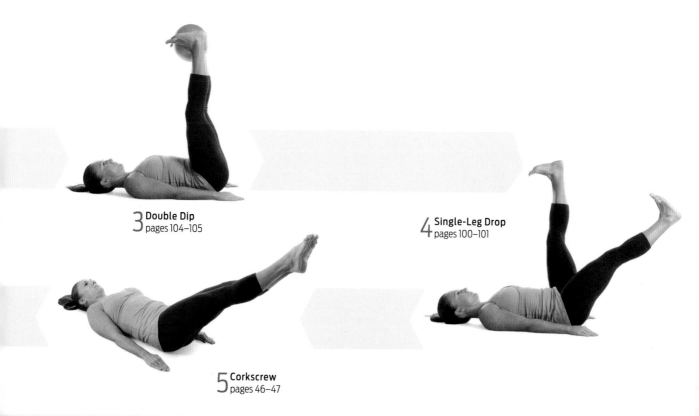

3 **Double Dip**
pages 104–105

4 **Single-Leg Drop**
pages 100–101

5 **Corkscrew**
pages 46–47

Leg Workout

Pilates is renowned for the lean, long lines it creates in the body. Nowhere is this more evident than in the results it achieves for legs. Follow this sequence of exercises to give your gams a rigorous yet gentle workout.

1 **One-Leg Circle**
pages 36–37

2 **Side Leg Kick**
pages 56–57

7 **Wide-Legged Plié**
pages 142–143

6 **Standing Leg Extension**
pages 144–145

The Arm Toner

The following exercises emphasize small, repetitive, and precise motion— all the better for achieving arms you won't be able to wait to show off.

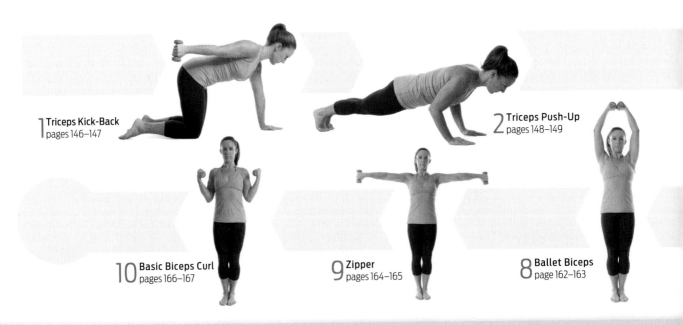

1 **Triceps Kick-Back**
pages 146–147

2 **Triceps Push-Up**
pages 148–149

10 **Basic Biceps Curl**
pages 166–167

9 **Zipper**
pages 164–165

8 **Ballet Biceps**
page 162–163

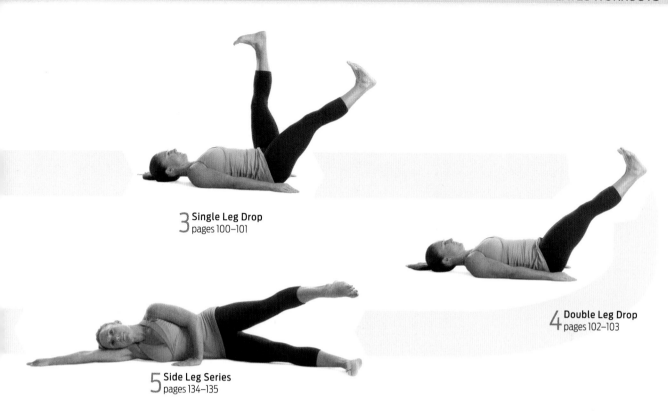

3 **Single Leg Drop**
pages 100–101

4 **Double Leg Drop**
pages 102–103

5 **Side Leg Series**
pages 134–135

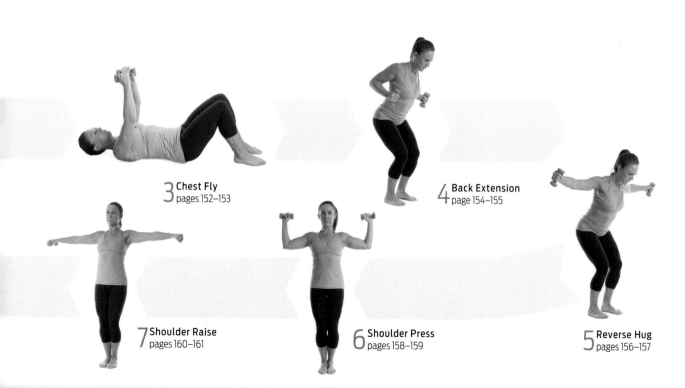

3 **Chest Fly**
pages 152–153

4 **Back Extension**
page 154–155

7 **Shoulder Raise**
pages 160–161

6 **Shoulder Press**
pages 158–159

5 **Reverse Hug**
pages 156–157

Spinal Call

This short sequence is great for energizing your body and mind any time during the day. Although it seems like the focus is on stretching and strengthening the spine, you'll also be working those abdominals as you support every movement along the way. Notice that you start and end with the same exercise—but see how different that exercise feels the second time around.

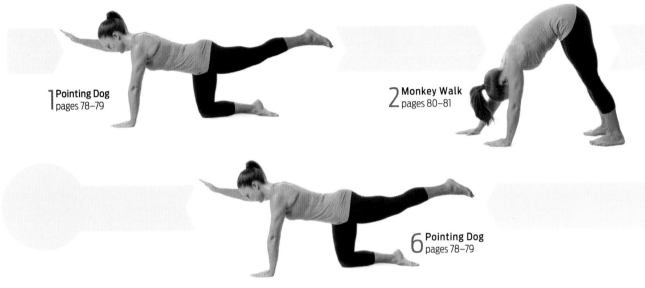

1 Pointing Dog
pages 78–79

2 Monkey Walk
pages 80–81

6 Pointing Dog
pages 78–79

Back Basics

When performed properly, the following workout will target your back without straining it. When working the back in Pilates, remember that less is more: some of the best back exercises involve keeping your spine and torso in place as you slowly and subtly move other parts of the body.

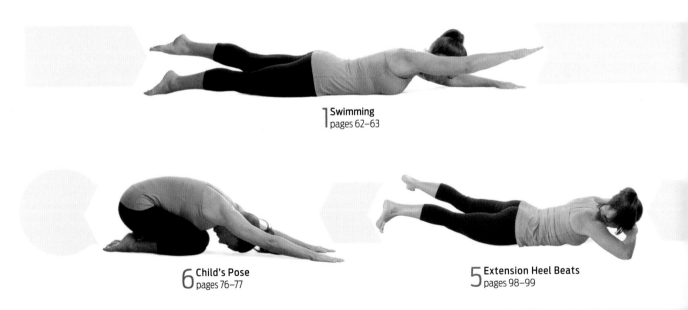

1 Swimming
pages 62–63

6 Child's Pose
pages 76–77

5 Extension Heel Beats
pages 98–99

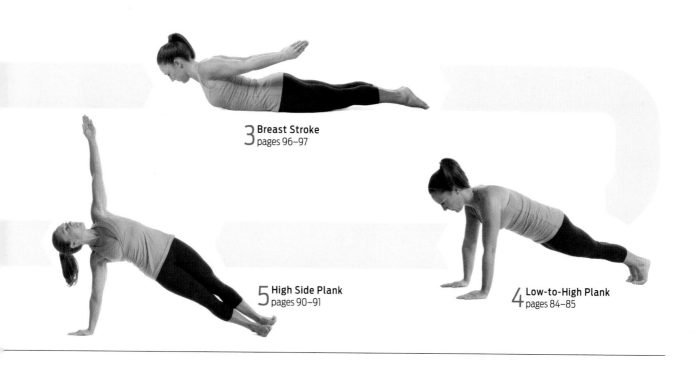

3 **Breast Stroke**
pages 96–97

5 **High Side Plank**
pages 90–91

4 **Low-to-High Plank**
pages 84–85

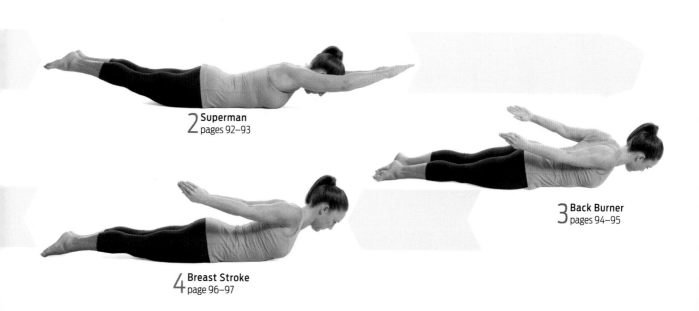

2 **Superman**
pages 92–93

3 **Back Burner**
pages 94–95

4 **Breast Stroke**
page 96–97

Target: Glutes

Strong glutes are key to a strong core, and the following sequence will really tone this muscle group. As a bonus, this sequence also works the hamstrings, abdominals, and back muscles.

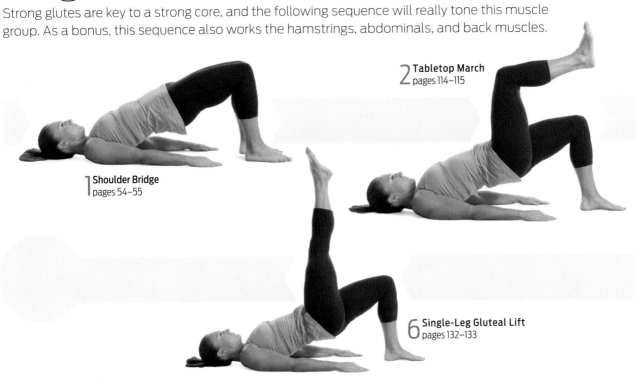

2 Tabletop March
pages 114–115

1 Shoulder Bridge
pages 54–55

6 Single-Leg Gluteal Lift
pages 132–133

Stretch Your Limits

Sometimes, at the end of a demanding workout (or simply a demanding day), our bodies cry out for a good stretch. The following exercises will do the trick. Complete just a few more repetitions or stay in the stretches a few moments longer than initially planned for a truly restorative session.

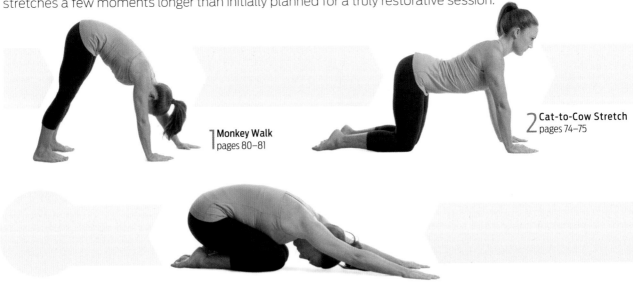

1 Monkey Walk
pages 80–81

2 Cat-to-Cow Stretch
pages 74–75

6 Child's Pose
pages 76–77

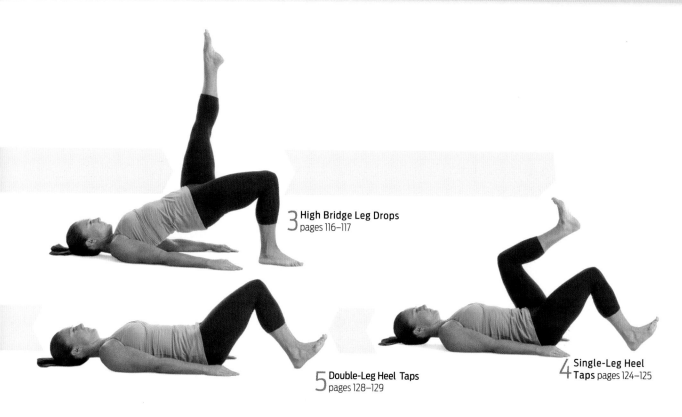

3 **High Bridge Leg Drops**
pages 116–117

5 **Double-Leg Heel Taps**
pages 128–129

4 **Single-Leg Heel Taps** pages 124–125

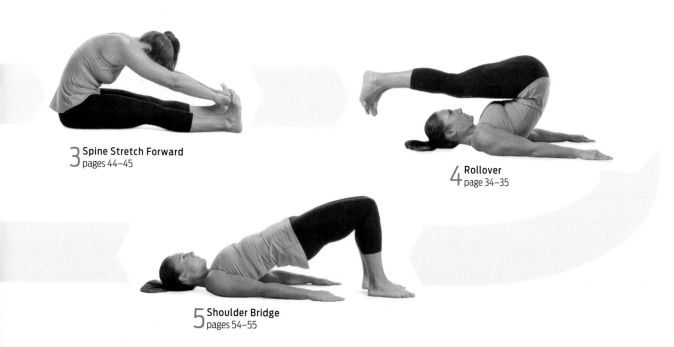

3 **Spine Stretch Forward**
pages 44–45

4 **Rollover**
page 34–35

5 **Shoulder Bridge**
pages 54–55

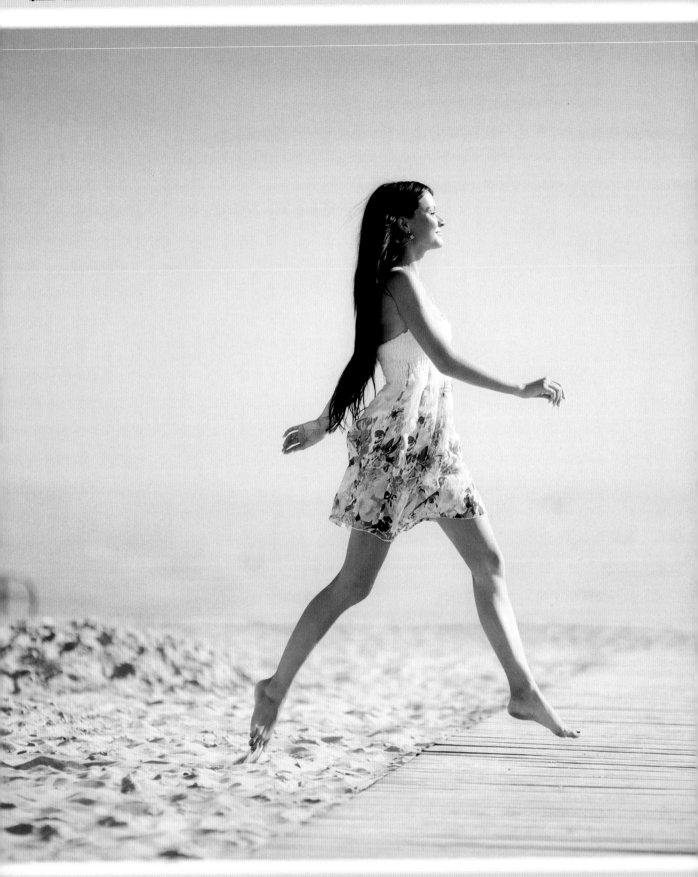

Conclusion

Through practicing these Pilates exercises—and, along the way, growing to understand the principles and physiology that underlie them—you are giving yourself a tool for lifelong well-being. As you've probably realized by now, Pilates gets your body moving . . . but it also does so much more. Regular practice connects you to your breath and challenges your powerhouse muscles, making you sleeker, tighter, and leaner so that you stand taller and feel stronger. While fine-tuning your arms, legs, and waistline, you are also tuning in to how your body functions as a unified whole.

The great thing about Pilates is that you can make it your own. Don't limit yourself to workouts suggested here: try mixing and matching, doing what feels right. Dip into these pages as you construct an exercise program that evolves with your needs. By exploring this book, you are well on your way to a practice that will benefit your body and mind for years to come.

Glossary

GENERAL TERMINOLOGY

abduction: Movement away from the body.

adduction: Movement toward the body.

alignment: In the yoga practice each pose has an ideal position of the body. If the body is in alignment, then it is placed in a proper way so that the muscles can work more effectively; they don't have to grip or struggle to hold the position, thus preventing injury. Each pose has its own alignment points, such as where to place the hands, feet, or torso, so learning a pose means also learning its proper points of alignment.

anterior: Located in the front.

cardiovascular exercise: Any exercise that increases the heart rate, making oxygen and nutrient-rich blood available to working muscles.

cardiovascular system: The circulatory system that distributes blood throughout the body, which includes the heart, lungs, arteries, veins, and capillaries.

c-curve: Describes the shape of the back and spine when the stomach is "scooped" inward and the muscles surrounding the spine are stretched.

cervical spine: The upper area of the spine immediately below the skull.

cool-down: A yoga pose performed at the end of the season the works to cool and relax the body after more vigorous exertion.

core: Refers to the deep muscle layers that lie close to the spine and provide structural support for the entire body. The core is divisible into two groups: major core and minor core muscles. The major muscles reside on the trunk and include the belly area and the mid and lower back. This area encompasses the pelvic floor muscles (levator ani, pubococcygeus, iliococcygeus, pubo-rectalis, and coccygeus), the abdominals (rectus abdominis, transversus abdominis, obliquus externus, and obliquus internus), the spinal extensors (multifidus spinae, erector spinae, splenius, longissimus thoracis, and semispinalis), and the diaphragm. The minor core muscles include the latissimus dorsi, gluteus maximus, and trapezius (upper, middle, and lower). These minor core muscles assist the major muscles when the body engages in activities or movements that require added stability.

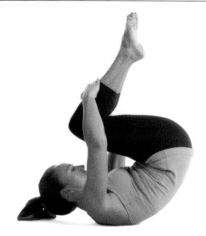

cueing. A Pilates teaching and learning tool, involving the use of descriptive, everyday images to stimulate correct practice.

diaphragm: A large dome-shaped sheet of muscle that sits beneath the lungs and extends across the bottom of the rib cage. Also known as the thoracic diagram.

diaphragmatic deep breathing: A technique that helps you maximize the benefits of your Pilates practice by fully utilizing your diaphragm.

extension: The act of straightening.

extensor muscle: A muscle serving to extend a body part away from the body.

external rotation: The act of moving a body part away from the center of the body.

fitness ball: A large, inflatable ball sometimes used for support during a Pilates workout that brings the core into play, using the powerhouse muscles for balance and stability. Sometimes called a Swiss ball.

fitness circle. A flexible ring, usually made of metal, with pliable handles, adds resistance to a Pilates movement when the sides of the circle are squeezed together. Also known as a Magic Circle.

flexion: The bending of a joint.

flexor muscle: A muscle that decreases the angle between two bones, as bending the arm at the elbow or raising the thigh toward the stomach.

foam roller: A foam rubber tube available in a variety of sizes, materials, and densities, which can be used for stretching, strengthening, balance training, stability training, and self-massage.

hand weights: Small weights that can be incorporated into Pilates exercises to enhance strengthening and toning benefits.

iliotibial band (ITB): A thick band of fibrous tissue that runs down the outside of the leg, beginning at the hip and extending to the outer side of the tibia just below the knee joint. The band functions in concert with several of the thigh muscles to provide stability to the outside of the knee joint.

imprinted position: A position in which the navel is pressed toward the spine, the lower-back muscles are lengthened and strengthened, and the abdominal wall is flattened.

internal rotation: The act of moving a body part toward the center of the body.

lateral: Located on, or extending toward, the outside.

lateral breathing: A breathing technique whereby the breath is directed into the sides and back of the rib cage.

lumbar spine: The lower part of the spine.

medial: Located on, or extending toward, the middle.

neutral: In Pilates, describes the position of the legs, pelvis, hips, or other part of the body that is neither arched nor curved forward.

neutral position: A position in which the natural curve of the spine is maintained, typically adopted when lying on one's back with one or both feet on the mat.

peeling the spine: Rolling the spine gradually up or down, vertebra by vertebra.

Pilates ball: A small inflatable ball, usually about 9 inches (23 cm) in diameter small ball that can be incorporated into a workout to enhance fitness benefits. For instance, when grasped between the knees, it helps to engage the hard-to-tone muscles of the inner thighs. Any small ball can achieve this effect.

Pilates mat. A firm mat, usually made of foam rubber, that is at least one-half inch (1.27 cm) thick. The roll-up variety typically measures about 72 to 86 inches (180–220 cm), with widths varying from 20 or so inches to close to 40 inches (50–100 cm).

Pilates Principles: Six principles considered to be essential to effective practice of Pilates, including centering, control, flow, breath, precision, and concentration. Some version of these principles is found in every Pilates style.

posterior: Located behind.

powerhouse: Refers to a group of strong muscles around the lumbar spine, extending from between the bottom of the ribs and the line across the hips into the arms and legs.

rotator muscle: One of a group of muscles that assist the rotation of a joint, such as the hip or the shoulder.

scapula: The protrusion of bone on the mid to upper back, also known as the "shoulder blade."

stacking: Aligning parts of the body, such as the hips, one on top of the other.

tabletop position: A position in which one lies on one's back with legs raised, knees bent at a 90-degree angle, and shins parallel to the mat.

thoracic spine: The middle part of the spine warm-up: Any form of light exercise of short duration that prepares the body for more intense exercises.

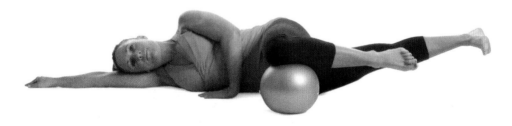

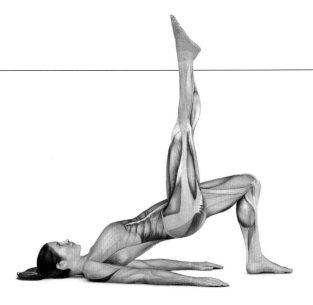

LATIN TERMINOLOGY

The following glossary list explains the Latin terminology used to describe the body's musculature. In some instance, certain words are derived from Greek, which is therein indicated.

Chest

coracobrachialis: Greek *korakoeidés*, "ravenlike," and *brachium*, "arm"

pectoralis (major and minor): *pectus*, "breast"

Abdomen

obliquus externus: *obliquus*, "slanting," and *externus*, "outward"

obliquus internus: *obliquus*, "slanting," and *internus*, "within"

rectus abdominis: *rego*, "straight, upright," and *abdomen*, "belly"

serratus anterior: *serra*, "saw," and *ante*, "before"

transversus abdominis: *transversus*, "athwart," and *abdomen*, "belly"

Neck

scalenus: Greek *skalénós*, "unequal"

semispinalis: *semi*, "half," and *spinae*, "spine"

splenius: Greek *spléníon*, "plaster, patch"

sternocleidomastoideus: Greek *stérnon*, "chest," Greek *kleís*, "key," and Greek *mastoeidés*, "breastlike"

Back

erector spinae: *erectus*, "straight," and *spina*, "thorn"

latissimus dorsi: *latus*, "wide," and *dorsum*, "back"

multifidus spinae: *multifid*, "to cut into divisions," and *spinae*, "spine"

quadratus lumborum: *quadratus*, "square, rectangular," and *lumbus*, "loin"

rhomboideus: Greek *rhembesthai*, "to spin"

trapezius: Greek *trapezion*, "small table"

Shoulders

deltoideus (anterior, medial, and posterior): Greek *deltoeidés*, "delta-shaped"

infraspinatus: *infra*, "under," and *spina*, "thorn"

levator scapulae: *levare*, "to raise," and *scapulae*, "shoulder [blades]"

subscapularis: *sub*, "below," and *scapulae*, "shoulder [blades]"

supraspinatus: *supra*, "above," and *spina*, "thorn"

teres (major and minor): *teres*, "rounded"

Upper arm

biceps brachii: *biceps*, "two-headed," and *brachium*, "arm"

brachialis: *brachium*, "arm"

triceps brachii: *triceps*, "three-headed," and *brachium*, "arm"

Lower arm

anconeus: Greek *anconad*, "elbow"

brachioradialis: *brachium*, "arm," and *radius*, "spoke"

extensor carpi radialis: *extendere*, "to extend," Greek *karpós*, "wrist," and *radius*, "spoke"

extensor digitorum: *extendere*, "to extend," and *digitus*, "finger, toe"

flexor carpi pollicis longus: *flectere*, "to bend," Greek *karpós*, "wrist," *pollicis*, "thumb," and *longus*, "long"

flexor carpi radialis: *flectere*, "to bend," Greek *karpós*, "wrist," and *radius*, "spoke"

flexor carpi ulnaris: *flectere*, "to bend," Greek *karpós*, "wrist," and *ulnaris*, "forearm"

flexor digitorum: *flectere*, "to bend," and *digitus*, "finger, toe"

palmaris longus: *palmaris*, "palm," and *longus*, "long"

pronator teres: *pronate*, "to rotate," and *teres*, "rounded.

Hips

gemellus (inferior and superior): *geminus*, "twin"

gluteus maximus: Greek *gloutós*, "rump," and *maximus*, "largest"

gluteus medius: Greek *gloutós*, "rump," and *medialis*, "middle"

gluteus minimus: Greek *gloutós*, "rump," and *minimus*, "smallest"

iliopsoas: *ilium*, "groin," and Greek *psoa*, "groin muscle"

iliacus: *ilium*, "groin"

obturator externus: *obturare*, "to block," and *externus*, "outward"

obturator internus: *obturare*, "to block," and *internus*, "within"

pectineus: *pectin*, "comb"

piriformis: *pirum*, "pear," and *forma*, "shape"

quadratus femoris: *quadratus*, "square, rectangular," and *femur*, "thigh"

Upper leg

adductor longus: *adducere*, "to contract," and *longus*, "long"

adductor magnus: *adducere*, "to contract," and *magnus*, "major"

biceps femoris: *biceps*, "two-headed," and *femur*, "thigh"

gracilis: *gracilis*, "slim, slender"

rectus femoris: *rego*, "straight, upright," and *femur*, "thigh"

sartorius: *sarcio*, "to patch" or "to repair"

semimembranosus: *semi*, "half," and *membrum*, "limb"

semitendinosus: *semi*, "half," and *tendo*, "tendon"

tensor fasciae latae: *tenere*, "to stretch," *fasciae*, "band," and *latae*, "laid down"

vastus intermedius: *vastus*, "immense, huge," and *intermedius*, "between"

vastus lateralis: *vastus*, "immense, huge," and *lateralis*, "side"

vastus medialis: *vastus*, "immense, huge," and *medialis*, "middle"

Lower leg

adductor digiti minimi: *adducere*, "to contract," *digitus*, "finger, toe," and minimum "smallest"

adductor hallucis: *adducere*, "to contract," and *hallex*, "big toe"

extensor digitorum: *extendere*, "to extend," and *digitus*, "finger, toe"

extensor hallucis: *extendere*, "to extend," and *hallex*, "big toe"

flexor digitorum: *flectere*, "to bend," and *digitus*, "finger, toe"

flexor hallucis: *flectere*, "to bend," and *hallex*, "big toe"

gastrocnemius: Greek *gastroknémía*, "calf [of the leg]"

peroneus: *peronei*, "of the fibula"

plantaris: *planta*, "the sole"

soleus: *solea*, "sandal"

tibialis anterior: *tibia*, "reed pipe," and *ante*, "before"

tibialis posterior: *tibia*, "reed pipe," and *posterus*, "coming after"

Icon Index

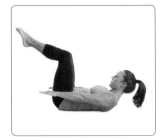

Hundred I
page 28

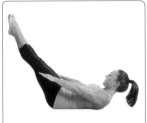

Hundred II
page 30

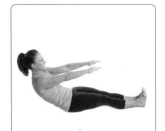

Roll-Up
page 32

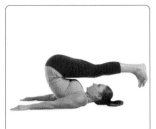

Rollover
page 34

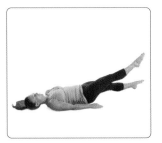

One-Leg Circle
page 36

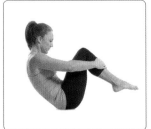

Rolling Like a Ball
page 38

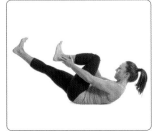

Single-Leg Stretch
page 40

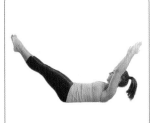

Double-Leg Stretch
page 42

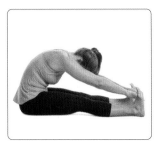

Spine Stretch Forward
page 44

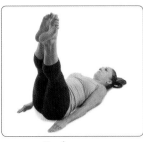

Corkscrew
page 46

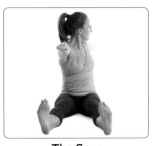

The Saw
page 48

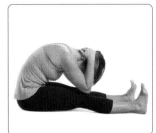

Neck Pull
page 50

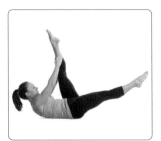

The Scissors
page 52

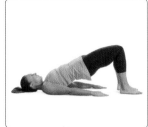

Shoulder Bridge
page 54

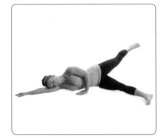

Side Leg Kick
page 56

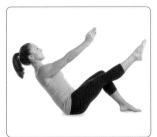

Teaser Prep
page 58

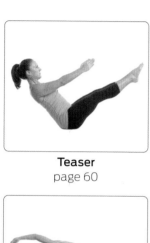

Teaser
page 60

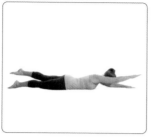

Swimming
page 62

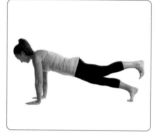

Leg Pull Front
page 64

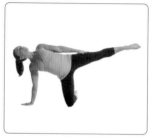

Side Leg Kick Kneeling
page 68

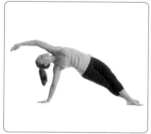

Side Bend
page 70

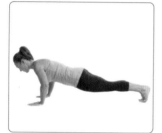

Push-Up
page 72

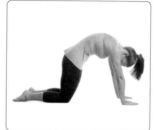

Cat-to-Cow Stretch
page 74

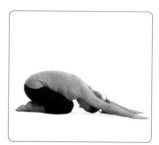

Child's Pose
page 76

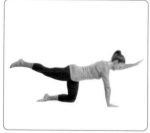

Pointing Dog
page 78

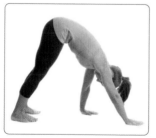

Monkey Walk
page 80

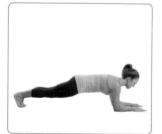

Low Plank
page 82

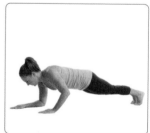

Low-to-High Plank
page 84

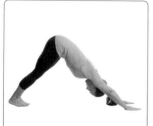

High Plank Pike
page 86

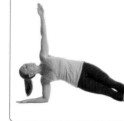

Low Side Plank
page 88

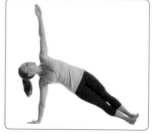

High Side Plank
page 90

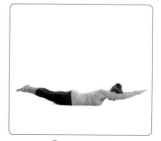

Superman
page 92

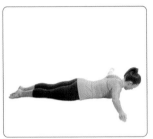

Back Burner
page 94

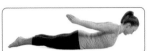

Breast Stroke
page 96

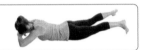

Extension Heel Beats
page 98

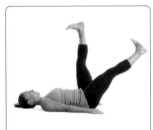

Single Leg Drop
page 100

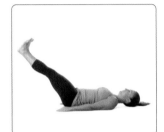

Double Leg Drop
page 102

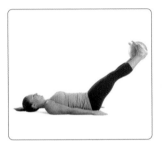

Double Dip
page 104

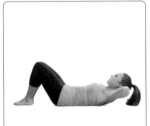

Basic Crunch
page 106

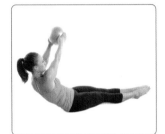

Figure 8
page 108

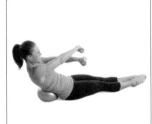

C-Curve Arm Cross
page 110

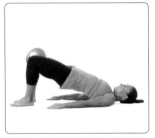

Pilates Ball Tabletop Bridge
page 112

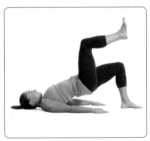

Tabletop March
page 114

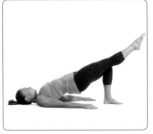

High Bridge Leg Drops
page 116

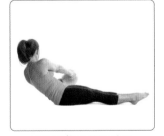

Waistline Warrior
page 118

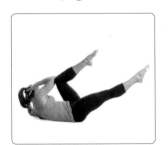

Bicycle Twist
page 120

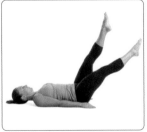

Criss-Cross
page 122

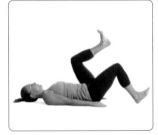

Single-Leg Heel Taps
page 124

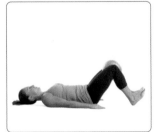

Pilates Ball Heel Taps
page 126

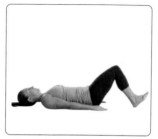

Double-Leg Heel Taps
page 128

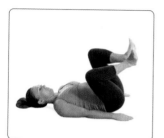

Frog
page 130

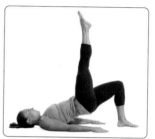

Single-Leg Gluteal Lift
page 132

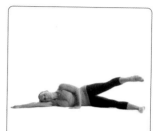

Side Leg Series
page 134

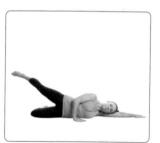

**Side-Lying Straight-
Leg Circles** page 136

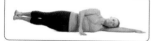

**Side-Lying Double-
Leg Lift** page 138

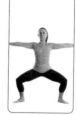
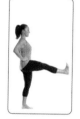

**Wide-
Legged Plié**
page 142

**Standing Leg
Extension**
page 144

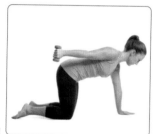

Triceps Kickback
page 146

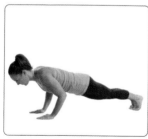

**Pilates Ball Side-Lying
Inner Thigh** page 140

Triceps Push-Up
page 148

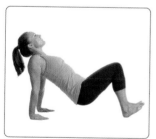

Triceps Dip
page 150

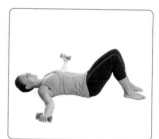

Chest Fly
page 152

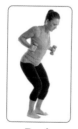
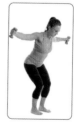

**Back
Extension**
page 154

**Reverse
Hug**
page 156

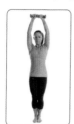
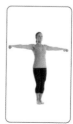

**Shoulder
Press**
page 158

**Shoulder
Raise**
page 160

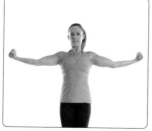

Ballet Biceps
page 162

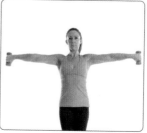

The Zipper
page 164

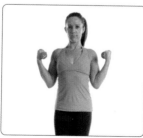

Basic Biceps Curl
page 166

About the author

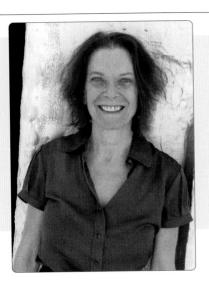

Isabel Eisen, a native New Yorker and trained dancer, lived and worked in Denmark for many years—first as a performer and then, increasingly, as an educator. She initiated and directed theater arts programs for adults and young people and was part of a group of British and Danish performing artists who established Scandinavian Theatre School in Copenhagen. She wrote a book, *Danseværksted*, and articles about her teaching ideas and practice, which were published in Denmark. Her deep involvement in teaching coupled with her interest in intelligent exercising, led her to Pilates, which she studied intensively for several years at Body Control and Stott Pilates studios in Denmark. In 2010, Ms. Eisen returned to New York City, where she continues to pursue her work with teaching, writing, and Pilates.

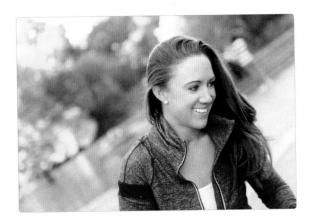

Pilates model and consultant Brooke Marrone turned her successful collegiate pursuits into a thriving full-time career as a fitness trainer. Her post-graduation experience studying under one of Boston's top trainers formed the basis for the safe and effective training philosophy that she follows today. In 2007, Brooke moved to New York City and started Brooke Marrone Fitness, a private, in-home training business. Brooke also hosts group classes in New York's Central Park and has been named an ambassador for Lululemon in both 2011 and 2012. Brooke's certifications include Personal Training, Pilates and Group Fitness. Brooke's training strategy is to stick to the basics while always trying to incorporate something new and unique into each workout. She integrates her personal training and Pilates knowledge to make each workout safe, creative, and challenging.

Credits

All photographs by Jonathan Conklin Photography, Inc., except for the following:

Page 9 top right Eponaleah/Shutterstock.com; page 10 Charles Masters/Shutterstock.com; page 11 top right Claudio Baldini/Shutterstock.com; page 16 middle Diana Taliun/Shutterstock.com; page 16 bottom right wavebreakmedia ltd/Shutterstock.com; page 17 top Venus Angel/Shutterstock.com; page 18 middle marcioalves/Shutterstock.com; page 18 bottom right FuzzBones/Shutterstock.com; page 20 middle left Caroline Eibl/Shutterstock.com; page 20 bottom left Beth Van Trees/Shutterstock.com; page 20 top right luchschen/Shutterstock.com; page 21 middle Zoom Team/Shutterstock.com; page 21 right Nyvlt-art/Shutterstock.com; page 22 top gresei/Shutterstock.com; page 22 bottom Zoom Team/Shutterstock.com; page 23 left Irina Tischenko/Shutterstock.com; page 23 top right Liliia Rudchenko/Shutterstock.com; page 23 bottom Zoom Team/Shutterstock.com; page 182–183 Ganna Malakhova/Shutterstock.com

All anatomical illustrations by Hector Aiza/3 D Labz Animation India, except the following:

Small insets and full-body anatomy pages 22–23 by Linda Bucklin/Shutterstock.com. Page 8 bottom by Leonello Calvetti/Shutterstock.com; page 14 Digital Storm/Shutterstock.com; page 15 right sam100/Shutterstock.com.